Hope Is the Thing

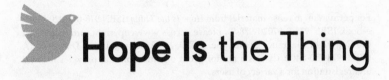

Hope Is the Thing

Wisconsinites on Perseverance in a Pandemic

Edited by
B. J. Hollars

WISCONSIN HISTORICAL SOCIETY PRESS

Published by the Wisconsin Historical Society Press
Publishers since 1855

The Wisconsin Historical Society helps people connect to the past by
collecting, preserving, and sharing stories. Founded in 1846, the Society
is one of the nation's finest historical institutions.
Join the Wisconsin Historical Society: wisconsinhistory.org/membership

Some pieces in this book were previously published on the Chippewa Valley
Writers Guild's "Hope Project" website. Additionally, several pieces appeared in
other media in slightly different forms: Araceli Esparza's on *Wisconsin Life*, John
Hildebrand's in *Local Lit*, Patti See's in the Eau Claire *Leader-Telegram*, and Jake
Wrasse's in *Volume One*.

The cover art, *We Get Through This Together* by Emily Maryniak, was created for
the Wisconsin Historical Society's COVID-19 Poster Project. Prints of the poster are
available to purchase through the Society's online store, shop.wisconsinhistory
.org/covid-19-poster-project.

Printed in the United States of America
Cover design by Emily Maryniak
Interior design and typesetting by Percolator Graphic Design

25 24 23 22 21   1 2 3 4 5

Library of Congress Cataloging-in-Publication Data

Names: Hollars, B. J., editor.
Title: Hope is the thing : Wisconsinites on perseverance in a pandemic / edited
   by B. J. Hollars.
Description: [Madison] : Wisconsin Historical Society Press, [2021]
Identifiers: LCCN 2021001163 (print) | LCCN 2021001164 (e-book) | ISBN
   9780870209772 (paperback) | ISBN 9780870209789 (epub)
Subjects: LCSH: COVID-19 Pandemic, 2020—Social aspects—Wisconsin. |
   Hope. | Wisconsin—Social conditions—21st century.
Classification: LCC HN79.W6 H56 2021 (print) | LCC HN79.W6 (e-book) | DDC
   362.1962/414009775—dc23
LC record available at https://lccn.loc.gov/2021001163
LC e-book record available at https://lccn.loc.gov/2021001164

For the bringers of hope,
and for those who shine it brightly.

"Hope" is the thing with feathers (314)

EMILY DICKINSON

"Hope" is the thing with feathers –
That perches in the soul –
And sings the tune without the words –
And never stops – at all –

And sweetest – in the Gale – is heard –
And sore must be the storm –
That could abash the little Bird
That kept so many warm –

I've heard it in the chillest land –
And on the strangest Sea –
Yet – never – in Extremity,
It asked a crumb – of me.

Contents

History isn't just in the past; it's happening every day. That's why in the course of its mission to collect, preserve, and share stories of our state's history, the Wisconsin Historical Society has often made efforts to document historic events as they occur. From journals kept by Civil War soldiers to photographs of the civil rights movement, these real-time collection efforts have resulted in valuable resources that provide vivid windows into significant events.

In early 2020, as a deadly virus made its way around the globe, it was evident that we were living through an extraordinary moment. The Wisconsin Historical Society put out a call for community members to participate in the COVID-19 Journal Project, which asked them to write about their experiences during the pandemic in journals to be donated to the Society's collections. Additionally, a number of Wisconsin artists contributed to the COVID-19 Poster Project, creating public information posters that could be used during the pandemic as well as by future generations. Such projects give Wisconsinites from all walks of life the opportunity to have their stories documented as part of our state's history.

When B. J. Hollars proposed this collection of writings in response to the pandemic, the Wisconsin Historical Society Press saw an opportunity to contribute to our agency's efforts to record history as it is happening. Hollars's project differed from the Society's other efforts in that he asked writers to reflect on a specific but universal topic: the myriad ways humans find hope in the face of strife. Hollars made a point of collecting pieces from different regions of the state, age groups, professions, and ethnic and religious backgrounds, efforts that aligned well with the Society's goals to share stories of all Wisconsin people, reflecting the diversity of our state.

While the writing of this collection's pieces was underway, the country faced another historic event, as the death of George Floyd in police custody led to nationwide protests and renewed discussions about police brutality against communities of color. Due to the timing, many of these pieces address the dual challenges of the pandemic and systemic racism, sometimes opining on topics that are sensitive, contentious, or political. These too are a reflection of our times.

In the interest of preserving the experiences and voices of this diverse group of writers, their pieces have been only minimally edited for style and clarity. We hope that in addition to being of interest and providing inspiration to contemporary audiences, these writings will serve as a vital part of a historical record: a snapshot in time of what people around Wisconsin were experiencing, thinking, and feeling during a difficult year.

Hope Is
One Foot in Front of the Other

B. J. HOLLARS

Shortly before sunrise, I strap my seven-month-old daughter into her stroller and take to the sidewalks around our western Wisconsin home. For three months now, this has become our ritual, our anchoring to the earth. We strike out for several miles, observing no humans, but instead, the natural world grown bold. And not just backyard critters. Sure, we see the squirrels and the rabbits, but some days we see deer, too, traipsing down the streets, bowing their heads between the neighbors' gardens. They sample all that has sprouted, chewing noisily before continuing their moveable feast.

If the deer see us, their recognition hardly registers. Perhaps they sense that we are no threat. Hope, for them, is a patch of fresh flowers and no one to shoo them away.

Hope, for me, is sharing with my daughter—who's been quarantined half her life—any glimpse of the world we can get.

Leaning low beside the stroller, I whisper the name of those creatures just ahead of us.

"Deer," I say. "Deer."

Her eyes widen, her world expands.

Sometimes hope is a humble thing.

The "Hope Project," too, was born humbly. It began one dismal day in March 2020 when, feeling hopeless myself, I called upon fellow writers to share with me where they were finding hope in the time of COVID-19. The call resulted in one hundred or so submissions, the majority of which were originally published on the Chippewa Valley Writers Guild's website. The guidelines were simple: each piece was limited to five hundred words

1

and with a title that broadly borrowed from Emily Dickinson's "'Hope' is the thing with feathers."

At the project's conception, it had no guiding principle other than my own need for hope. A month later, when stumbling upon the words of Maxine Hong Kingston, that guiding principle became clear. Kingston's words served as the directive I'd been looking for: "In a time of destruction," she remarked, "create something."

And create we did.

Today, I'm pleased to share with you the fruits of our labor: one hundred explorations of hope courtesy of writers throughout the state. Some contributors are seasoned authors; others are making their publication debut. Some are octogenarians; one is in middle school. They are racially diverse, geographically diverse, culturally diverse, and, I hope, representative of a cross section of our citizenry. In curating this work, my editorial philosophy centered on elevating and amplifying a range of voices to more fully capture this unprecedented moment.

Collectively, this work is meant to serve as both snapshot and time capsule, documenting the many unexpected places where hope has resided in the midst of this health crisis and beyond. Some contributors address the pandemic directly; others, more obliquely. Some pieces were written in the early days of the pandemic and reflect the uncertainty of that time; others were written several months deep and reflect our evolving understanding of our changing world.

While this project was born beneath the shroud of a virus, it ended up reflecting all the challenges our nation faced in the first half of 2020, none of which was more significant than the killing of George Floyd, which occurred less than a month before this writing. While I will never fully understand the pain endured by Black, Brown, and Indigenous people, many of our contributors do. And they write about that pain—and the occasional hope that springs forth—with such eloquence and force as to ensure that none of us will ever forget.

2

To view our country's health problems and racial problems as separate and distinct risks missing the larger point. Though they may be rooted in different places, our progress on both fronts is directly linked to human action. What we do or don't do in this moment means the difference between life and death, between freedom and oppression.

And hope alone is not nearly enough to solve these dual crises.

Having spent the last several months engaged with the subject of hope, I've reached a conclusion that "glass-half-full Hollars" never saw coming. While I'd previously believed hope to be the buoy that lifts all spirits, I now see its darker side.

Too often, hope is a telescope when what we need is a rocket ship.

By which I mean: hope alone won't take us where we want to go, but it can show us the way. Envisioning that destination is the first step toward reaching it—not that our state or country has any one destination in mind.

Wherever we end up, may the road be paved in justice. And may the view ahead be better than the one behind.

All of which brings us back to my daughter, the deer, and our morning constitutionals. Lately, we've been venturing further, and as our miles increase, so too, do our interactions. By sunup, the wildlife begins to give way to our fellow humans, most of whom walk alone or in pairs, and many of whom are masked. Under such conditions, I can't see their smiles, but I can feel them. We demonstrate our affection for one another by other means, most notably, the wide berths that have now become so commonplace, steering ourselves from the sidewalks like some terrestrial version of synchronized swimming. None of us needs to say anything for our message to be clear. By way of our detouring, we are telegraphing empathy, acknowledging shared responsibility, and reaffirming humanity, too.

Sometimes even the humblest actions are hopeful.

One morning, as a walker and I engaged in the awkward who-goes-which-way shuffle, we both found ourselves laughing at an experience that seemed equal parts necessary and absurd. Eventually, the walker and I worked out the details—she went left, we went right—and then, we both continued on our way. But before she was out of sight, I turned the stroller around so my daughter could get a quick look at the creature who had just passed us.

"Person," I said. "Person."

We continued on, one foot in front of the other, moving toward that better world.

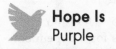 **Hope Is**
Purple

JIM ALF

Isolation with time on one's hands is for the imaginative the Club Sega Arcade of mental games. It is a factory for fancies. It is the breeding ground for hopeless despair. In such situations, thoughts formed whole from the detritus of splintered observations congeal into mirages too horrid to exist anywhere but the desert of phantasmal imagery. A favorite feeding ground for those thoughts is a buffet of physical signs and symptoms.

My symptoms were few, but signs were posted with regularity (remember that word) along the road to the most dangerous of destinations: self-diagnosis. That repeated sign was the gradual lack of need for the most hoarded, most fought over, decidedly topmost item on the list of civilized necessities in a pandemic of viral death threats: that soft, white squeezable roll of paper hung by the throne. That observation, with some unusual weight loss and lessened appetite morphed easily into dark suspicions of impending decline of health, surgery and debilitation, and eventual memorial service with a bluegrass band playing "I'll Fly Away" and friends' maudlin recitations of what a jolly good fellow he was before he flew away. Morbid thought is like yeast, expanding beautifully but full of gaseous bubbles, an apt metaphor because that was my only production. Surely my primary physician would sound alarms, begin testing, and schedule treatments, probably too late. She brushed me off.

I had talked on the phone to the clinic receptionist. She passed me on to a nurse who noted my medical complaint and said she would talk to the doctor. I asked for a test kit by mail. I was certain such dire observations would result in a call from the doctor posthaste. The nurse called. The doctor says if it gets worse, call in a few days. From the mortician's? Hope evaporated like a raindrop in Death Valley.

Phone calls apprised next of kin, powers of attorney were reviewed, obituary was updated, and plans for a dependent formed. What else was needed? Downsize now! Too late. Let the survivors do it. Goodwill can bring a truck. Then, what luck: I was notified my annual checkup at the VA was two days away and the doctor would call at 8 a.m. on Friday. On Friday, the day of fish fries, baked potato, and slaw, I didn't dare eat. I could only hope that phone call would be in time. It was.

The call was three minutes early, fortuitous because every minute counted. I had my list of symptoms ready, blood pressure and pulse taken. Fear billowed like a cloud. I recited my list. He asked if I had pain. No pain. Bloating? None. Itch all over? Never heard of it. "Drink plenty of prune juice," he said.

I had an unopened jug in the fridge. Hope came in a tall glass and was purple, cold, and tasty. Efficient, too. The treatment took ten minutes; later the cure lasted ten more. The call to reserve a full order of fish, five minutes. Hope survives, banishes fear, lights the way. Life goes on.

Jim Alf is a retired lumber sawyer, over-the-road truck driver, and author of *When the Ferries Still Ran*, a book of local history. He resides in Eau Claire.

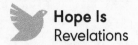

Hope Is
Revelations

ABAYOMI ANIMASHAUN

On the day and time
Of the passing of man

Pots and kettles
Will reconcile

Each will welcome
The other's black

From the same gourd
They'll drink wine

And from the same bowl
They'll eat yams

Feeding each other gently
In soft stewed mounds

*

Hens will borrow the moon's abacus
And take it to the coop

But just because
They borrow its abacus

Doesn't mean
They'll sing of the moon

They'll pull the beads
And sing instead

Of raised and feathered necks
Breeze beneath the cypress

And of love between gators
Octopi and ferrets—

Those gained and others
Unrequited

*

Goats will get drunk
On beer carefully brewed

To turn cheeks red
Or gently rouge

And warm from days
Of song and drink

Mugs raised
To nanny-goats

In blouse
And skirts trimmed

They'll raise their legs
In beat and rhyme

To tunes that echoed
From old men's hearts

On the day and time
Of the passing of man

Abayomi Animashaun is the author of three poetry collections and the editor of three anthologies. He teaches at the University of Wisconsin-Oshkosh and lives in Green Bay.

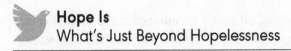

Hope Is
What's Just Beyond Hopelessness

JERRY APPS

With World War II ending in 1945, veterans returning home and rationing gone, we all hoped for better days ahead. As a twelve-year-old kid growing up on a central Wisconsin farm, I hoped for a better time than what we experienced during the dreaded war years with the many fears and sacrifices. Less than two years later, my personal hopes came crashing down.

One afternoon in January 1947, when I was in eighth grade at the Chain O'Lake one-room country school, I came home not feeling well. My mother, fearing I was coming down with a cold, sent me to bed early that evening—excused from doing my expected chores. It was not a cold. It was polio, a disease that spread rapidly from 1945 to 1955 throughout the country, until a vaccine became available.

Within a few days, my right knee was paralyzed and I was unable to walk, attend school, or do much of anything. For me, all hope had disappeared as quickly as one might blow out a candle. For days I was confined to a cot near the woodstove; we had no central heating, indoor plumbing, or electricity at the time. After six weeks or so, the disease's symptoms mostly disappeared, but polio left me unable to walk. With my dad's daily massaging of my bum knee with horse liniment—his answer to many health problems—I was able to walk, but not without a limp. Running remained a challenge. I returned to school in April and graduated eighth grade that spring.

In the fall I entered Wild Rose High School. All freshmen boys were encouraged, indeed expected, to take part in sports: baseball in the fall, basketball during the winter, and baseball again in spring. My bad leg eliminated me from all sports. Never in my young life had I felt more hopeless, bordering on worthless. But a couple of my teachers saw something in me that I didn't. The basketball coach encouraged me to announce the games over the gym's speaker system. The business teacher suggested I take a typing class. Once I got past the "only girls take typing" attitude prevalent at that time, I found I really enjoyed it. I had been milking cows by hand so had strong fingers, necessary for operating a manual typewriter, an L. C. Smith as I recall. The typing class produced the *Rosebud*, the high school's newspaper. Not only was I learning typing, I was learning how to write news stories. By the time I was a senior, I was editor of the newspaper, writing many of the articles, all of the editorials, and having a good time doing it. Slowly my feeling of utter despair and hopelessness was turning to hope.

When people ask me today where I learned to use a microphone and why I am a writer, I often answer with one word, *polio*. I am living, walking proof that something valuable can come from something difficult. Even knowing that, overcoming hopelessness with hope is not easy. I'm still working on it.

Jerry Apps, born and raised on a Wisconsin farm, is professor emeritus at the University of Wisconsin–Madison and the author of more than thirty-five books, many of them on rural history and country life.

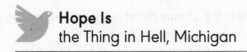

Hope Is
the Thing in Hell, Michigan

JODIE ARNOLD

Hell, Michigan, is an unincorporated community with a whopping three business fronts and a population of seventy-two people. And I was mayor for one day. Yes, you read that correctly. I was mayor of Hell for one day.

Let's back up a minute.

I just had one of those "quarantine birthdays," and honestly, I didn't mind. I'm forty-one years old. All I really wanted for my birthday was to drink before noon and not clean the house, which is coincidentally what I've been doing a lot since March.

In pre-COVID times, my fiancé had purchased my "mayor of Hell for a day" birthday gift with the intentions of us actually visiting there. Then he looked at the prices for flights and pretty soon abandoned that idea. I was left with an extremely socially distanced mayoral term and a huge package of unusual Hell-themed merchandise, including legal ownership of one-square-foot of Hell (I even got dirt), a coffee mug, and devil's horns. I wasn't really sure what it all meant.

As my one-day term began, he casually mentioned to me, "I think they might be calling you a few times today or something?"

The first call from Tristan came during the morning. "What in the hell have you been doing all morning?" she shouted at me before following up with, "I heard it's your damn birthday and you're mayor of Hell for the day, so let's get this swearing in ceremony over." We went through whatever one does to become Hell's mayor and then she said, "Your accent . . . are you from Wisconsin?"

It turns out Tristan has family from all over Wisconsin. She loves Point Beer. She's been to Chippewa Falls. We talked about the Midwest and the general weirdness of life right now. At some point, it stopped being a funny call about some temporary mayoral gimmick, and we just started talking.

Tristan has been out of work since March 26, work being running the tourism of a place like Hell, Michigan. You can imagine with a name like that, people from all over want to come for at least the magnet and photo next to the town sign. She's been trying to figure out unemployment but couldn't get an answer. She told me she had to keep coming to work because otherwise it would all go away, and then what would happen to the town? She owed it to people like me to make the most of my day in Hell.

Her entire day was committed to harassing me with phone calls, demanding me to make laws for the town (I decreed the town could drink only Busch Light, and that was a problem, as it should be), and eventually having me impeached around 6 p.m. She was getting paid for none of this, and that was not lost on me.

After my impeachment, Tristan gave me tips on a cheap way to get to Hell. (The jokes write themselves, folks.) I promised we'd visit. She said she'll always be there.

Jodie Arnold is from Stanley, Wisconsin, and currently resides in Chippewa Falls. She writes plays, creative nonfiction, radio dramas, and poetry and has performed as a featured storyteller for several regional events.

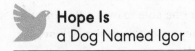

Hope Is
a Dog Named Igor

SHARON AUBERLE

It's a dismal morning here, though there's peace in this place where I write. At least until I look at the news. But for now, I'll drink my coffee, read good poems, and keep on. I'll listen to Rachmaninoff, feel the sun warm on my neck, taste fresh-baked bread. For now that's all I can do. Except, perhaps, pray. And wait for Igor to appear.

Igor is a dog of the Borzoi breed. And he is magical. He's also respectful and gentle, as this majestic Russian breed is described. Igor belongs to the neighbors up the road. His white coat is long and silky, with a golden collar at his throat. His hair flies in the wind as he dances through the yard with every bit as much grace as Baryshnikov.

Sometimes Igor will inch close and peer in the window. He seems curious, though it has taken months for him to venture so near the house. I am thrilled but know I must not startle him, only remain still and content with what he will allow. A warm feeling steals over me that he is not really of this world but only visiting, answering this mortal's troubled call. An angel, perhaps, in dog robes. For a moment our eyes lock and there is such intelligence and heart in his. I fall headlong in love.

On days when I fight to remain hopeful and positive in the midst of this raging pandemic, I think of Igor. He has given me a mantra to whisper sometimes, to shout other times: *When this is over . . . When this is over . . .*

I will find a rescue Borzoi dog.

I tell myself this again and again. In doing so, I'm acknowledging that yes, one day this terrible time will be over. I believe myself. Realistically, I may never be able to own a Borzoi; still, hope and possibility remain. They are out there somewhere, like Igor, reappearing when I need them most.

Sharon Auberle is a poet and photographer who served as Door County poet laureate from 2017 to 2019. She has authored a number of books, including her most recent, *Dovetail*, co-authored with Jeanie Tomasko.

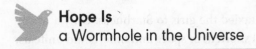

Hope Is
a Wormhole in the Universe

LAURA JEAN BAKER

Every pandemic requires a convincing argument, so this is what I tell myself as my husband, Ryan, and I dovetail at the kitchen sink. I am forearms deep in Palmolive suds. He is pantomiming flourishes of optimism, twirling the dry towel. Time has dilated and sucked us into a theoretical existence. Before COVID-19, we lived separately on the spacetime continuum of our everyday lives. Now we are metrics in Einstein's field equations for gravity, cocooned in a worm-tunnel of love.

Since 1996, Ryan and I have navigated distances far longer than the stretch of a collapsible tape measure, used once by a seamstress to pattern my wedding dress, five times by a midwife to chart the bubble of my fundus. For four years and six months, we studied in separate cities, Ryan rock-steady in La Crosse while I sojourned to Boulder, Madison, Buenos Aires, Madrid, and back again. I'd often fall ill, homesick for my partner in crime. Longing for Ryan felt like a virus.

Marriage in 2001 delivered us to a shared domicile in Ann Arbor, but graduate school was ruthless as a melon baller, scooping out my insides. Ryan was living; I was just a hollow pumpkin earning a creative writing degree.

By 2003, I'd recovered from my MFA, but then Ryan started law school. Everybody refers to law students' partners as widows for a reason. Our lawyers-in-training curled cadaverous over books in far-flung libraries, earning their Juris Doctorates while we stayed home. In 2004, our first daughter was born, followed by a brood of siblings in '06, '08, '10, and '13. As I breastfed on demand, Ryan and I didn't often sleep in the same bed. We dreamed and woke six billion light-years apart.

Before March 2020, on any given day, Ryan drove the boys to hockey; I drove the girls to music lessons. Or I chauffeured the boys to movies; he taxied the girls to Starbucks. Only a wormhole, a hypothetical shortcut in space and time, could unite us. "See you in fifteen years," we'd say.

Then on March 12, the University of Wisconsin–Oshkosh announced I'd begin teaching my English courses online, and ten days later, on March 22, the Wisconsin Supreme Court suspended in-person proceedings statewide. Slowly but predictably, everything closed, even the YMCA, our central hub for kids' activities. We stopped forcing our cars to guzzle gasoline, and we all decelerated.

"Hey, you," I said as if to a stranger in a cafe. I winked, and he smiled. This was our corona-inspired meet-cute.

Against the backdrop of our own fear and vigilance, amid our children's frustration and noise, Ryan and I had suddenly been thrust together again. We synced our lives, recalibrated our designs on togetherness, began walking five laps a day—one for each child—around the mile-long neighborhood circle.

Governor Evers's stay-at-home order has allowed us to merge with propulsive force. Despite all the dangers a wormhole presents—exotic matter, radiation, the threat of collapse—it's unexpectedly radiant in here.

Laura Jean Baker is the author of *The Motherhood Affidavits* and associate professor of English at the University of Wisconsin–Oshkosh. She is working hard to be optimistic, #safeathome with her husband and five children.

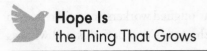

Hope Is
the Thing That Grows

MEREDITH BALL

After a week of social distancing, I'm feeling the need to be alone. Having three children means that social distance equals family togetherness—a lot of family togetherness. And so, I go on runs. I run in the rain with a hat pulled over my face, and I run when the freeze returns. But the best runs are the ones when the sunlight warms the air I breathe and the ground beneath my feet.

On this day, the sun is out in full force. I head toward campus, and as I close in on the dorms, I see parents moving their children out of their rooms. It wasn't so long ago that my own parents did the same for me. Back then, it seemed so chaotic—the hustle and bustle of fathers steering minivans toward the spots closest to the door, while mothers snagged the nearest empty cart and began piling high suitcases, duffels, and dirty rugs.

But today, everything is subdued. Only a few families are present, and none of them are wasting time with chaos. They don't smile, they don't socialize, they just get the job done. A few months back, when this ritual was repeated in reverse, nobody could have predicted a college year ending like this—in March, and at a distance of six feet away.

As I continue running through campus, I'm reminded of a more recent past: freshly planted bulbs placed into the dirt by the soon-to-be furloughed groundskeepers. Those tulips and daffodils should have been for the college students, enticing them outside after another long Wisconsin winter. They should have born witness to new friendships, flirting, and the emergence of new people blossoming before their petaled eyes. Instead, they're stuck with the occasional wayward runner like me.

Still, the first blooms give me hope. Hope that one day soon those students will return to their friendships, their flirting, their blossoming. And that the furloughed workers, too, will return to their jobs. And hopefully, the tulips and daffodils will witness it all.

Finishing my run, I see my own children playing in our yard. And I know that this time—this virus—will change them, too. They won't get to finish second grade or kindergarten. They, too, are losing their rites of passage. But like the spring flowers, there is growth here. After this season of turmoil, they will emerge from the soil anew, ready to take on the world.

Meredith Ball is a mom, teacher, and wife living in western Wisconsin. She enjoys running, reading, and being with her family (but maybe not this much).

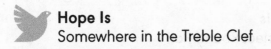

Hope Is
Somewhere in the Treble Clef

AVIROOP BASU

Hope is somewhere in the treble clef
Somewhere between the tall grass and blue skies of Telemann
In the dark gray clouds of Shostakovich
Between tales of Valkyries and Nutcrackers—
A thoughtful first movement
A peaceful fourth.

Like a hand tugging you up
After a fall
Scraped and injured
I trudge on
I simply hold the neck
Orient my shoulder
And let the melody free.

When the world is in disarray
Small strokes of the bow
Coupled with effortless vibrato
Is all it takes to wash my strife away.

Aviroop Basu, a student in Eau Claire, wrote this while attending Delong Middle School. His hobbies include martial arts, violin, and tennis.

19

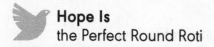

Hope Is
the Perfect Round Roti

LOPAMUDRA BASU

Hope is the thing that you can roll into a dough, press with your fingers, pummel with your palms, and transform with the addition of dried fungus into a loaf of bread. And yet this simple staple vanished from grocery aisles as most of the country came under shelter-in-place orders. The essential ingredient needed for bread—active dry yeast—also disappeared. This sparked the new quest for breads without yeast, and the sourdough emerged as the favored choice, the result of many hours of nurture from the creation of a fermented starter to the full glory of the boule. However, I found myself traveling an opposite course; instead of perfecting the sourdough, I sought the unleavened humble *chapati* or *roti* of my youth in India.

The *chapati* evokes mixed emotions. The *roti* baked in earthen tandoors seduced me during my college years in Delhi. *Rotis, naans, kulchas,* and *parathas,* the resplendent variety of Indian flatbreads with their aroma of buttery *ghee* and herbs wafting from so many roadside eateries. Many migrant workers in the city work in these *dhabas* and contribute to the economy of Indian cities. Many of them work as domestic help rolling out fluffy *chapatis* for urban upper-middle-class homes. In North America, I have resolutely rejected the labor of the Indian flatbread, making do with ready-made tortillas of the local grocery or vacuum-packed bags of Indian *chapatis*, which always leave a little longing on my palate.

As the bread shortages generated a plethora of photos of homemade sourdoughs, I got to work on whole wheat flour and a little warm water. The trick is to pour a little water at a time and knead till a firm and pliable dough emerges. Allow the dough to rest for thirty minutes before breaking it into small balls and using a floured rolling pin to shape each ball into a circle. Next, on a hot griddle, each rolled out flatbread has to be dry roasted and pressed till it fluffs up, full of air. There are many chances of failure in this project. The dough might be sticky, the rotis may not rise, but the hope for the perfect round and fluffy roti lives on.

My family appreciates my imperfect rectangular *chapatis*. As we eat our lentils and *rotis*, we feel a sense of powerlessness in the face of the global pandemic. In India, where our parents are sheltering in place, the lockdown has forced millions of migrant workers to walk thousands of miles to their villages, without the hope of a single *chapati* and sometimes without water. We live with the niggling worry for our elderly parents, but what is that in comparison to the grief of those who died trying to walk to their homes? We find groups in Delhi serving meals to stranded migrants and wire them money. But it is in the act of rolling my *chapati* that I feel the greatest bond with invisible labor, and in fluffing a perfect flatbread, the hope of human survival.

Lopamudra Basu is professor of English at the University of Wisconsin-Stout and lives in Eau Claire, with her husband and son.

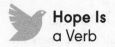

Hope Is
a Verb

EMILY BERTHOLF

Hope is a million tiny things we use to prop ourselves up and propel ourselves forward through times that feel distant and strange.

Week one: My teenaged children sleep in on mornings that unfurl from a long weekend to a longer spring break. Each closed in their rooms with their music and screens, social distancing seems natural to them. My husband, deemed essential, goes to work as usual. I navigate working remotely and repainting our bathroom walls an off-white shade ironically named Social Butterfly. The smell of paint reminds me of my dad. Creedence Clearwater Revival, Pat Benatar, and Tracy Chapman blare from my phone. Suddenly, I'm twelve again, painting a room in my parents' cellar Ballet Pink, transforming the dark, cobwebbed room into a dance studio. "See, Dad, not bad," I say out loud when I'm done, wishing he could see it. Seventy-four with emphysema, he's the reason we're staying home.

Week four: My youngest son plops next to me as I drink my morning coffee. Bursting from the quiet days of learning at home, he discloses stories of the playground and classrooms he won't admit he misses.

Week six: Two cardinals build a nest in the bush outside my window. Down the block, a neighbor puts a garden fence around a fallen female robin and her nestling huddled in the grass. I wonder if other birds come to help the mom feed her nestless nestling so she doesn't have to leave it alone. My children patter around the house, between the kitchen and in and out of their rooms, chatting with each other and their friends deep into the night.

Week eight: We walk to my parents' house on Mother's Day. My son sets a Tupperware box filled with homemade cupcakes he baked and decorated on the front stoop and knocks. We wait on the sidewalk. When my parents open the front door, we wave, smile, and blow kisses in the air.

Week twelve: I hear about a Black Lives Matter protest from a coworker. We're phasing into reopening. When I get home from work, my children ask if we can go. We don masks and join hundreds of Black, Latinx, and white families, couples, neighbors, and people of all ages walking through the streets where I grew up, where I've raised my children. We move and shout along to the young leader's call and response: "No Justice, No Peace." "Black Lives Matter." Off to the side, a young Black family watches the moving crowd with their daughters. The youngest girl sits in a stroller in front of her mother. The other little girl holds her father's hand. She looks to be about six, the same age Ruby Bridges was in 1960.

Maybe hope isn't a thing at all. Let hope not be a thing, a noun. Let hope be a verb, an action, a movement, a promise we intend to keep.

Emily Bertholf is a writer from Milwaukee, where she resides with her family. Her stories and poems have appeared or are upcoming in several anthologies.

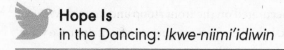

Hope Is
in the Dancing: *Ikwe-niimi'idiwin*

KIMBERLY BLAESER

They died within days of one another on White Earth Reservation: the aunties I never knew, Naomie and Edith, victims of a late wave of the Spanish flu. At the kitchen table where our hands peeled apples, shelled peas, or cleaned rice, my mother would recall the story her own mother told:

> The sisters fell ill together. School-aged Naomie longed to see the Christmas pageant she now could not be a part of. From her bed, she pleaded to watch from a safe distance—"jist through the window." Pomp of the pageant, however, went on without her. Edith passed; and Naomie, who declared she did not want to live without her, followed her baby sister in that sad December.

All this is legend—the exact details of that era swallowed by family truth. I do not know the numbers who died in the village of Nay-tah-waush or who else in my extended family fell ill but survived. I do know the deaths haunted. My grandma's next daughter, born in 1931, carried the legacy of both lost girls in her name: Naomi Edith Antell. When the 2020 spread of coronavirus reached Wisconsin, I lived at first in the fever shadow of old losses.

However, another legacy of Spanish flu on Great Lakes Ojibwe reservations continues today—the Jingle Dress Dance. When the father of an ill young girl prayed for her healing, the regalia we still fashion and the dance we continue to perform came to him in a dream. Following his vision, women created dresses adorned with metal cones that "sing" with the dancer's moves. When four women performed the ceremony, the story says the sounds called the young girl back. Growing stronger throughout the night, she finally joined the dancers.

Anishinaabe people believe in the Jingle Dress tradition as healing for spirit and flesh. When the pandemic hit one hundred years after the Spanish flu, several Native friends and I found hope in performing this symbolic dance. Connecting by Facebook, Instagram, text, and e-mail, we grew our sacred circle. Soon women across the continent joined in virtual ceremony—University of Wisconsin–Milwaukee colleagues, cousins in California, a former student in Walpole Island First Nation, White Earth friends, a fellow writer in Illinois—hundreds, all dancing for our ailing world.

Each Saturday, we gathered our regalia—moccasins, hair adornments, feather fans, and the ancient medicine dress, *zaangwewemagooday*. In our sheltering, we danced in March snow, in April by overflowing rivers and ponds, on porches when it rained. Spirits that move through the air, words and ancient rhythms of songs, motion of our bodies, the tinkling of the cones coming together, and our memory of survival across generations soothed us.

As the weeks passed, my daughter arrived home from college. Now before our dancing, our hands smooth and plait hair or tie one another's belts; after our dancing as we rest on the sunny hillside, I tell her the stories. I share legends old and new of illness, hope, and healing—of *Ikwe-niimi'idiwin*, the women's dance.

Kimberly Blaeser, past Wisconsin poet laureate, has published five poetry collections. An Anishinaabe activist and environmentalist from White Earth Reservation in Minnesota, Blaeser is a professor at UW–Milwaukee and MFA faculty member for the Institute of American Indian Arts in Santa Fe.

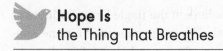

Hope Is
the Thing That Breathes

PEGGY BLOMENBERG

I hold my breath, waiting for the sound of my newborn taking her very first breath. She breathes! and cries—and I cry, too, in great exhausted jubilation at her shocked announcement of life. Simultaneously with breath, her voice is born, borne on that very first exhalation. Our cheers, laughter, and tears applaud her brand-new breathing—robust and sure, as practiced as if she has been doing it all her life.

Still, many nights I steal to her crib to look for the rise and fall of that impossibly tiny chest, then expel my own held breath in relief and gratitude.

Life: in-breath, out-breath, repeat. Precious, fragile, infinitely dear.

Decades later, in 2016, I sit stunned with this all-grown-up daughter at the bedside of her husband, who collapsed at work and was found not breathing. He is thirty-five. We are in Neuro-ICU. A ventilator breathes for him, buying time, keeping our hope alive minute by minute. As long as breath follows breath, we can hope for recovery.

As a singer, I know that breathing, so life giving and seemingly so natural, can be improved upon. I recently attended a master class in singing in which the professor demonstrated for her student singers how to better hold their bodies to make a space for the air, enabling the deep and effective breathing that is foundational for excellent singing. It was a marvel, the difference in the sound that emerged from these already fine singers as they allowed their breath to effortlessly become their song.

Our first breath and our last breath pretty much delimit life as we know it outside the womb. In between, in daily routines, we might stand up and go for "a breath of fresh air." Or take a break to "catch our breath." We have a sudden inspiration (literally, in-breath) that "breathes new life" into stale patterns or ideas. Celebrating special occasions, we expand our lungs to the max, blowing up balloons, blowing out candles, making joyful noises. (Well, not so much right now, but we can hope.) Swimming, we dive deep then race back to the surface for air. Hiking at altitude, our breathing becomes more rapid the higher we go. Very thin air and thin ice are both dangerous in that they do not fully support us.

The last breath, for many, comes too soon. To our grief, my son-in-law did not recover. But it was not for lack of a ventilator. Simply, he had been without oxygen for too long before being found, resulting in irrecoverable brain injury. For many in communities around the world, right now, the availability of such a machine—to buy time, offer hope, and provide support through the critical period—is the difference between recovery and death. I hope that we will each do our part to delay transmission and thereby spread the serious cases out over time, so that those whose survival depends on such machines may hope for recovery.

Peggy Blomenberg is a hopeful, grateful, and mostly positive person who has worked as an editor and educator. Farm-raised in Indiana, she has lived in Wisconsin's Chippewa Valley since 2009.

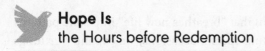

Hope Is
the Hours before Redemption

TIM BRENNAN

in the field, a hundred
or so
Canada geese congregate,
maybe they are praying—
they think not of social distancing,
think not of previous loved ones.
they don't seem sad,
seem not to think about dying,
maybe not to think enough is enough
for them—
but each time they migrate, they quiet their wings,
write in haiku the understanding of the seasons.

Tim Brennan is a former Altoona, Wisconsin, resident and UW–Eau Claire graduate whose poetry has appeared in several publications and whose one-act plays have been performed across the United States.

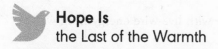

Hope Is
the Last of the Warmth

RYAN BROWNE

The first week Dean came to the farmers market in McPike Park on the near-east side of Madison, he wore his black mask and stood an appropriate six feet away.

I had seen him many times in the taproom, always seated at the bar, always bending one ear or another, sometimes mine, though I had the cover of owner-type concerns to steal away under. Our bartenders, on the other hand, were exactly where they ought to be, and Dean seemed to treasure that, his eyes big under a mop of sandy blond hair, with the joviality of someone laughing through the telling of a joke at a table of friends.

The farmers market, where my tent was staked in place for three hours, was now a critical tent pole in our operations—preselling beer for pickup across the street at our taproom, which had been closed since March 15, 2020. That's when Working Draft Beer Company, which I'd cofounded just two years prior, dropped to zero revenue overnight.

Shortly after, I had to inform nineteen of twenty team members we no longer had a job for them.

Then there were the calculations of debt, not to expand or amplify the heartbeats of our new business but to triage, stop the hemorrhaging, because the heart cannot be amputated to save the rest of the body.

Then there was the task of restarting the business. We had to rethink our whole way of doing business over a weekend, switching from face-to-face service to e-commerce. Then, we had to do it again. Suddenly everything that was Working Draft had to fit inside a sixteen-ounce can.

Then, like a cat chasing a laser pointer, we faced the moving target of when to safely reopen a taproom that had been banging every Friday and Saturday with live-wire energy from wall to muraled wall.

Today, the taproom is a half-lit carcass of quadruple-stacked chairs collecting grain dust, upside-down tables, uprooted couches and lounge seats, blown-out speakers, pallets of crowlers, vacant tap lists, and empty barstools.

That first week at the farmers market, I was not prepared for Dean to stay as long as he did. For close to two hours, he moved from topic to topic: beer styles, beer brands, breweries, of course, but also his living situation, an old drafty house owned by his family and former commune members, as well as his new apartment off Atwood behind Alchemy bar, built so snug to the tracks that passing trains rattled everything he owned.

Despite his consuming presence beside the tent, Dean was also hyperaware of other guests walking up to the tent. He'd clip his comment when necessary, allowing me to do whatever business I could.

Then he'd resume.

The next week, he returned with a camping chair so he could continue to discuss a range of topics with me: his "mental breakdown," his interest in sword fighting and live dueling, his favorite fantasy authors and series and the intricacies of their worlds blended with the renderings of magic, the weather.

I nodded. I agreed. I *huh*-ed and mindlessly drifted through the market, meandering among stalls. It was either go through the motions or collapse inward, ruminating on the Jenga tower of stress my presence at this market represented.

One week, as Dean packed up, the sun was setting, red and mottled like one of the two suns of Tatooine. Wildfires were carrying ash this far north, he noted. For a stretch of time I didn't bother to note, didn't even consider noting, we looked at the setting sun together, silently.

And for weeks, I sat in the park at the market with Dean and listened to where he'd like to live in the world, what he knew about exotic barley varieties, his thoughts on the gentrification of East Madison as a lifelong eastside resident and East High grad, his eventual plans to brew mead and its future variants and adjuncts.

And for weeks, after taking orders for beers to-go, Dean and I enjoyed the sunsets together, each one arriving sooner than the last, each one radiant, romantic in a way, because of the quiet affection Dean and I shared for those moments.

The last week Dean and I sat together, the sun began to set over the skyline, shining bright and below the tent overhang at a steep fall angle. The light was warm, and I rolled my back to it. But Dean didn't, allowing it to laser-beam across his eyes. He basked in that fading light, soaking up as much as he could.

Ryan Browne is a poet and co-owner of Working Draft Beer Company in Madison.

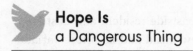
Hope Is
a Dangerous Thing

NICKOLAS BUTLER

My son and I donned our masks and left our rural property
south of Eau Claire for the first time in three weeks. We had finally eaten through just about every calorie of fresh food in our
refrigerator, right down to our last onion and sad-looking lime;
it was time to buy groceries.

Both of us had looked forward to this expedition, stir-crazy
as we were. But as we drove closer to the city, the amount of
traffic around our vehicle disconcerted me. The last time I'd left
the house, I was struck by how our community had resembled a
ghost town: closed businesses, empty roads, no pedestrians. But
today, the world appeared normal.

At the grocery store, my son and I seemed to be in the minority
of shoppers wearing masks. As we piled food in our cart, I was
filled with an increasing sense of dread. I understand that a mask
may or may not prevent someone from contracting COVID-19,
and yet, it doesn't seem like a bad idea either. It is a conservative
gesture, like hedging one's bets, like a small discomfort to ensure
the freedoms of my fellow citizens. After a half hour of shopping,
I was very ready to return to my home. I think this sense of disappointment and dread no doubt contributed to one of the more
expensive grocery bills I've ever seen.

It was difficult to not link today's unmasked faces and heavy
traffic with last night, when the Wisconsin Supreme Court struck
down Governor Tony Evers's stay-at-home order, a preventative
measure supported by 70 percent of polled Wisconsinites—no
doubt worried for their own health or the health of a vulnerable
loved one in this uncertain and dangerous time. News reports
published photographs of Wisconsin taverns filled with patrons.
Because, you know, who demonstrates more judicious behavior

than a drunk person filled with pent-up longing and perhaps a dash of wanton disregard for public health?

I wish that I could write an essay filled with optimism, perhaps illustrating the hope I normally identify with migratory birds, the first brave vernal tulips, or the new apple blossoms on my property. But I don't feel hopeful, and maybe right now, hope is an empty promise, an emotion that prevents us from acting rationally, scientifically. One thing that has disappointed me during this crisis is how predictably the situation was politicized, dividing our country and state, rather than unifying a citizenry hungry for facts, informed leadership, and let's face it—hope. Instead, two defining philosophies arose: caution informed by science and medicine, and a reckless opposition prizing the almighty dollar and perceived personal freedom. Middle ground was few and far between.

What I want more than anything these days is not more emotion, not more optimism in the face of such a little-known and deadly virus. What I want is science, medicine, and a smart plan. Without a plan, how can there be optimism?

At the moment, I identify less with Emily Dickinson and more with Lana Del Rey, who sang, "Hope is a dangerous thing for a woman like me to have."

Nickolas Butler is the internationally best-selling and prize-winning author of *Shotgun Lovesongs*, *Beneath the Bonfire*, *The Hearts of Men*, *Little Faith*, and *Godspeed*. He lives south of Eau Claire with his wife and their two children.

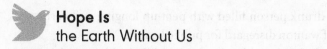

Hope Is
the Earth Without Us

BRENDA CÁRDENAS

Without Us

Hope is teosinte, maize's ancestor,
planting itself in our garden,
reaching all the way up to the rain
gutter, stalk so tall, I could climb
it like a ladder to the roof. In silent
Chicago streets, hope listens
to robin's yeep, cardinal's whistle.

It is the River Thames flowing clean
and green through London fog,
the twelve-lane LA sky clear of smog,
fish flashing their silvery fins
as they swim in Venice's cloudy canals
turned turquoise aquariums, swans
floating on their glassy surfaces.

Hope swings with monkeys on ropes
from ledges to balconies, seizing a town
hall in Thailand; spins with sheep
on an empty playground's roundabout;
spots goats and peacocks strutting
down the thoroughfares of Wales, wild
boar ransacking Barcelona, and coyotes

crossing the deserted Golden Gate.
Hope is nilgai strolling roads in Noida,
olive ridley turtles free to lay eggs
on Odisha's beach without tourists

swarming for snapshots. Hope is a family
of red fox emerging from bushes
to sun themselves in the parking lot

outside our window. Capitalism's
induced coma quiets the hum
of vibrations in the Earth's crust—
the planet's seismic noise on hold
while we quarantine to escape microbes
that look like sea urchins or allium
flowers. Soon, trickster teosinte—

grain of the gods—will push
past our first floor reminding us
that ancestors float on wind, return
in beaks of birds, in the busy hands
of squirrels digging and tilling the good
Earth that will make its own medicine,
cleanse itself, and keep turning, long

after our flames have blown out.

Brenda Cárdenas is the author of *Boomerang* and three chapbooks and
has coedited or had work appear in numerous other collections. Cárdenas has served as the Milwaukee poet laureate and teaches at the University of Wisconsin–Milwaukee.

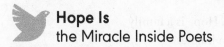

Hope Is
the Miracle Inside Poets

FABU PHILLIS CARTER

The poem "'Hope' is the thing with feathers" is framed in my home as a daily reminder that the existence of hope in the United States, especially in historically perilous times, is truly a miracle. It was a miracle for hope to exist in the poetry of Emily Dickinson, and it is even more of a miracle for hope to exist in the poetry of African American women.

Dickinson was a single woman dependent upon her family for every critical resource because she was unmarried when women were either economically tied to their husbands or male relatives. By 1861, when it is believed that she wrote the poem, even a free-born African American woman had a different, more limited reality than hers. White women abolitionists, inspired by the cruelty of slavery to fight to end the system of owning human beings, also began to recognize that they were in a type of bondage too.

Slavery ended in 1865, yet African American women continue to struggle with both racism and sexism. African American women, never a subset of history, or "her story," in the United States, took their destinies into their own hands from their arrival in this country. Since they were equal to men in the oppression they suffered, they resisted slavery with a passion equal to African American men. They also fought for a hope that included everyone in their actions and in their words.

As early as 1845, poet, writer, journalist, and activist Frances Ellen Watkins Harper, the only child of free African American parents, published her first collection of poetry. By 1854, her second collection of poetry was published. It ended up being reprinted twenty times. Harper had a prolific career emphasizing hope as both a woman and as an African American. While both Harper and Dickinson are parts of my legacy as a woman poet,

I have to call on Harper's life and writings to keep hope alive in my own work.

While the status of all women has improved, as an African American woman poet, I still fight the dual oppressions of racism and sexism. In 2020, with the advent of the COVID-19 pandemic coupled with deadly inequalities in the United States, ranging from health inequalities to racially motivated murders, not nearly enough has changed. Every day I read the framed words of Dickinson in my home and think of Harper's struggle to be free. I embrace the hope both wrote about, still perched, that refuses to die in either my poetry or in my life. Hope is a miracle inside poets.

Fabu Phillis Carter is a working Wisconsin poet and was Madison poet laureate from 2008 to 2012. She has published seven books and enjoys giving guest lectures, leading workshops, and doing poetry readings and storytelling events for children.

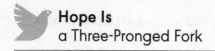

Hope Is
a Three-Pronged Fork

JUSTIN CARTER

On Easter Sunday, Erica Barnard reached for her phone and connected to the livestream of our morning church service. She was attending virtually, not only for pandemic purposes but because she was confined to her hospital bed. Erica had advanced liver disease, and this would be her first time gathering with a community of believers in at least two decades. On Easter, we reflected on the sacred cry of our suffering Savior, "*Eli, Eli lema sabachthani.*" Erica spontaneously shared her own reflection and typed in the chat, "Being forsaken is a powerful emotion." In those few words, we learned a lot about Erica's life.

Days later, I had the opportunity to have a conversation with Erica over the phone as she revealed to me the renewal of her faith. Erica continued to join our services through a screen, in sickness and in health, as a faithful bride to Christ. The only Sundays she ever missed were when she was on a ventilator.

In her final weeks I learned about a tattoo that she, her mom, and sister had planned to get on Mother's Day. Earlier in the year, Erica had seen a social media post about a young girl with a terminal illness who had told her pastor that she wanted to be buried with a dessert fork. Why? Because while clearing the evening meal, the girl's wise grandmother had whispered, "Keep your fork because the best is yet to come."

Believing that the best was yet to come for herself as well, Erica wanted to capture this story with a tattoo. The fork would be the dinglehopper from *The Little Mermaid* with the grandmother's wise words inscribed below. The tattoo was never inked.

Erica is no longer waiting for dessert, and her anticipation for the "best to come" is now realized. After her funeral, her mother handed me a three-pronged fork in memory of her daughter.

I keep it on my office bulletin board, held by a single thumbtack pressed between a pair of silver prongs. The fork looks as if it may fall at any moment, yet somehow it never does. Every day, as I begin my pastoral work, I catch a glimpse of Erica's fork on the bulletin board. It reminds me that even in adversity, and even while walking in the valley of the shadow of death, hope prevailith much.

Justin Carter is a follower of Jesus, married to his high school sweetheart Renee, and they have four children. He is the lead minister of Cornerstone Christian Church in western Wisconsin.

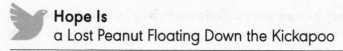

Hope Is
a Lost Peanut Floating Down the Kickapoo

MATT CASHION

Hope? You want hope? I'm usually a cup's-half-full kind of guy, but through the first half of 2020, just days before the deadline my overly hopeful editor imposed for this assignment, my cup was not only empty, it was missing.

Heather and I loaded our kayaks and drove to Vernon County to look for it. We stayed overnight with our friends Jean and Terry (greeted them while wearing masks, then maintained our distances) on their forty-acre homestead so we could get up early and follow them and their canoe down the narrow and sandy roads that wound through the Driftless region of south-western Wisconsin toward the slow-moving Kickapoo.

Edith—Jean and Terry's six-year-old granddaughter who had also stayed the night—woke early, checked the chicken pen for eggs (two), then returned, eager for conversation and an-swers to long lists of impossible questions. I'm not a morning person. We don't have children. This kind of energy was one reason why. Edith urged her grandpa to watch her jump on his trampoline. I urged him to make coffee. "I'll watch you," I said, and off we went. She bounced while hugging her stuffed horse, and I sat on a nearby lawn mower, gripped the wheel, and pre-tended to race away.

"It doesn't work," she said.

"Why did the chicken cross the road?" I asked.

She recited the obvious. I dug deeper, searching for philo-sophical truth. "But *why*?"

"To get to the orchestra," she said.

"Yes."

"And to go to church," she said.

"To join the chicken choir and play saxophone," I offered.

"And to go to McDonald's."

"For french fries."

"And arugula."

"Yes."

"And to get away from the coyote's shadow," she said.

I paused. "Do you think a coyote would eat a cat?"

"No," Edith said. "Too many ticks."

She climbed down and ran to the chicken pen, as if worried for their safety. I followed the leader. She pointed to each of the six hens and taught me their names. "Luke," for example. "Luna." I forget the rest.

"Hold this." She handed me her stuffed horse, entered the pen, squatted, flapped her arms, and made chicken sounds. I made chicken sounds too. We laughed at each other.

Later, the water took us beside ancient rock cliffs topped with cloud-high pines. I remembered how small I was, how young. Just fifty-two. We coasted beneath bridges where hundreds of barn swallows sprang from nests and swarmed in circles because we were trespassing. We moved through this primitive and quiet place that cradled the sun, a sanctuary that has weathered floods and droughts and will continue to endure.

Situated between her grandparents in their canoe, Edith turned to face her grandpa. She pulled out a bag of snacks. From my trailing kayak, I asked what she was eating.

"Peanuts," she yelled. "I'm putting one in the water so it will float to you."

The current took it the opposite way.

"Thank you," I said, cup found. Full.

Matt Cashion teaches creative writing and literature at the University of Wisconsin–La Crosse and has published a short story collection and two novels. Born in North Carolina and raised in Georgia, he has enjoyed calling La Crosse home since 2006.

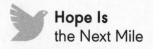

Hope Is
the Next Mile

ERIN CELELLO

I used to be a distance athlete. Marathons and halves, century rides, and Ironmans. Now, my knees are bone on bone, and with two young boys, there's little time to train. But the mental gymnastics—to keep yourself moving forward, to keep from falling in a heap, curled in on yourself with agony—are well ingrained after all these years. And chief among them is this: do not look too far ahead.

If, at the start of an endurance race, you were to anticipate each tick of the hours ahead—every step until the finish, the toenails you'd lose and the patches of skin that will be burned or rubbed raw by the end—you might never begin. So, you focus on your stride. Your breathing. That telephone pole up ahead. When the next aid station is. You keep things small, because small things are doable.

Before one marathon for which I was particularly anxious, my father-in-law imparted four words to me: *anything for a mile.* During that race, those words were sometimes a heartbeat. Others, a pounding drum. At one point, when the bursa in my hip got next-level angry and my run became a hobble, they were a silent, primal scream. But always, they were true.

When the world stopped on Friday, March 13, when our jobs went online, when our kids' schools went virtual, when overnight I became a kindergarten and second grade teacher, an art, physical education, and music teacher, a librarian and a cook in addition to a college professor, when the network talking heads marinated in fear and numbers—lack of protective equipment and ICU capacity and positive cases and deaths—I couldn't seem to catch my breath. And alone in my car, I cried. Because it seemed too much. To absorb. To understand. To do. To feel.

Anything for a mile.

Those words returned, fitting, and still true. My body remembered; so did my mind. It centered, went small. A pile of groceries to sanitize meant we had food. The breath of warm wind meant spring, and then summer. The laughter of my children, the crush of their little bodies against mine, their arms around my neck, meant that right here, right now, things were okay.

When will there be a cure? Will we go back to school? When will life go back to normal?

No one knows, I tell my boys when they ask these questions, and point out all the small, good things around us instead: green grass, downy goslings, air vibrating with the bass of marsh toads, legs that run and lungs that breathe, unbidden time together.

It's hard to do much beyond this. The numbers are too big. The future too uncertain. The end of the day is a sufficient goalpost for now.

So, while we wait for the world to right itself, we keep things small. We keep on. But we dream, too—about smiles, unmasked. Laughter without a screen between. Hugs and touch and togetherness.

While we wait, we hope, for these simple things to start again.

Erin Celello is a Madison-based essayist and author of two novels, *Miracle Beach* and *Learning to Stay*. She is an assistant professor at the University of Wisconsin-Whitewater and Drexel University's MFA program.

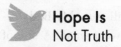

Hope Is
Not Truth

DOROTHY CHAN

Here's a metaphor for you: Hope was the name of a Ty Beanie Baby I owned when I was a kid. You might remember the Beanie Babies craze of the nineties, also known as the economic bubble that lured consumers into buying every one of these six-dollar floppy animals they could get their hands on. Toy stores would limit the amount of Beanie Babies each family could buy in one trip. A couple in Las Vegas even took their collection to divorce court. And why? Ty Warner, the creator of these "collector's items," somehow convinced America that Beanie Babies would someday be worth "thousands," even teasing out early retirement dates. But in reality, Ty had factories all over China making thousands and thousands more of Patti the Platypus, Legs the Frog, Goldie the Goldfish, and yes, Hope the Bear.

I got rid of my Beanie Babies collection a long time ago, but to this day, nineties kids visit their parents' homes over the holidays and find these stacks of nostalgia. These stacks of nostalgia once promised us the "hope" that they'd be worth thousands, helping us with college debts, rent payments, etc. And now, these stacks of nostalgia are piling up in unsold eBay listings. Go to almost any flea market or second-hand store, and you'll find Beanie Babies.

It was all a false hope, after all. It almost felt too easy, didn't it? I guess that's why economic bubbles happen. We want an easy solution. But also, capitalistic crazes are very harmful.

I'm taking us on this walk down nineties memory lane to say the following: hope is not truth. Truth is at our very core, and we may search for it endlessly.

I believe that it is understandably human nature to hold onto a glimmer of hope in almost every situation. I brought up the Beanie Babies saga because I've had lots of consecutive sleepless nights, where I go into deep internet dives, studying human nature. This Ty story is also grounded in the dangers of hive mind mentality.

That being said, I think it is very easy to ask people to have hope. But I also do not believe in an easy solution, especially during a time like this. Rather, I believe in a solution that is grounded in truth, confrontation—and yes, even pain.

It takes a lot of strength and truth for me to say that I have not been feeling hopeful. It's not my goal to feel negative, either. But I think it's also completely realistic to lose hope during times like this. I also have to point out that my response is also beyond just me and my own internal thoughts. But then what am I left with? I am left with truth.

When I think about truth, I think about Truth with a capital *T*. I remember how my mentor, Lyrae Van Clief-Stefanon, used to tell us during undergraduate workshop, "In poetry, we want to seek the truth with a capital *T*." I'll remember these words forever.

Dorothy Chan is an assistant professor of English at the University of Wisconsin–Eau Claire. She is the author of *Revenge of the Asian Woman* and *Attack of the Fifty-Foot Centerfold*.

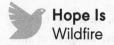

Hope Is
Wildfire

DEKILA CHUNGYALPA

If there is one truth COVID-19 has exposed, it is that our neoliberal economic system is, by design, a pyramid scheme, which leaves the marginalized—Black, Indigenous, people of color, women, the working class, the poor—holding the bag. From on top of their pyramids, the pharaohs who thrive on throwaway culture now demand their sacrifices in the form of throwaway people. Those who work service jobs, blue-collar jobs, and who can't work from home have been made essential and redundant all at once. It has taken a few decades to get here: reorganizing us into echo chambers, bartering our loyalty to corporations and political parties for a semblance of belonging, distracting us from understanding that we are unmoored by our individualism and unprotected in our isolation.

We might have gone along with it. It is possible the pandemic by itself would keep us in a frozen paroxysm of waiting. Maybe if there had been some physical manifestation of mourning from our country's leaders of our dead—ten thousand, fifty thousand, one hundred thousand, and still counting—we would have taken a deep shivering breath and settled down. But in a world where demagogues and dictators feel threatened by the expression of collective grief, our collective suffering can be suppressed only so much. George Floyd. Breonna Taylor. Ahmaud Arbery. Unlike other instances when African Americans have been killed and brutally oppressed through police-sanctioned violence in the United States, people of other races are suddenly, painfully realizing they also are George, they also are Breonna, they also are Ahmaud. Those who are subjugated by a system that puts a boot on their neck while demanding they pull themselves up by their bootstraps have woken up.

Meanwhile we are also living through probably the hottest year in human history. January was the hottest January in recorded history. So were April and May. Our fossil-fuel-dependent economies are creating more climate-related disasters and more devastation around the world to be borne yet again by the marginalized. Everything is interconnected; you cannot care about humans and ignore climate change; you cannot care about climate change and ignore race; you cannot care about race and ignore politics; you cannot care about politics and ignore humans. And vice versa. Maybe this is how a society learns empathy—through shared suffering. Maybe this is when non-Black races acknowledge the systemic racism that entraps Black people in America and uphold that Black lives matter as much as their own. Maybe white people will realize once and for all that economic systems that benefit them but create misery for others are inherently unstable and therefore unsustainable.

Hope is a wildfire that needs to breathe, dance, and burn. It needs to be fed with possibilities so that healthy ecosystems can be born anew. Hope is fearsome. It cannot be bought, it cannot be forced, it is not easily contained. Hope fills pharaohs, demagogues, and dictators with trepidation. I burn with hope. We burn with hope. What else can explain this civil rights uprising, nurtured everywhere by resolute Black women leaders, spreading like wildfire, in all fifty US states, in hundreds of US cities, and in more than seventy countries? It is long past time for America to be born anew.

Dekila Chungyalpa is the director of the Loka Initiative, an environmental education and outreach platform for faith and indigenous leaders, at the University of Wisconsin–Madison. Her areas of expertise include community-based conservation, climate resilience and preparedness, spiritual ecology, and faith-led initiatives.

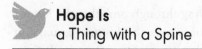
Hope Is
a Thing with a Spine

CHRISTINA CLANCY

A few years ago, Elizabeth Kolbert visited Madison to promote her book *The Sixth Extinction*. She discussed with a packed house the startling ways in which human beings are "reorganizing the biosphere," from climate change's impacts on plant and animal habitats to the distressing problems with the world's oceans. The news was grim, and she delivered it like an oncologist sharing a poor prognosis with a worried patient.

A young parent in the audience raised her hand. "But what should I tell my kids?" she asked. "This is all so . . . depressing."

Kolbert was thoughtful but stone-faced. What she said in response stuck with me, and I found myself returning to her statement again and again during the long, angsty days of lockdown. Essentially, Kolbert said that there is no reason for parents to believe—or expect—that our children will have easier lives than our own. In fact, she said they'll likely face a barrage of severe challenges to their health and environment, and that parents would be well served to teach their children to be resourceful and resilient. In essence, she had no patience for sadness, a useless emotion in the face of crisis.

And then that crisis happened. My own kids, now grown, ended up back at home again in Madison once the pandemic hit. My son was yanked from his study abroad program in Greece and was trapped for five hours in a long line at O'Hare after the abruptly issued travel ban, a true superspreading event. My daughter, a recent college graduate, had just started her first "real job" and was having a hard time adjusting to working from home. Like most everyone, we lived without schedules or structure and watched the news obsessively. As hard as it was for parents with young kids to be stuck in quarantine together, at least the little ones were still young and oblivious. It seemed

almost harder to watch my adult children register the serious-
ness and enormity of the social, economic, and political challenges we faced, grapple with the implications for their future,
and sort through the frustrating ambiguity of the crisis.

Like the mother at that event, I didn't want my kids to be sad.
But Kolbert's advice echoed in my head. She was right that this
was likely the first crisis of many they would face, and it was
better to address it head-on and develop the coping skills they
needed to deal with adversity instead of wallow in despair. Hope,
for me, came from not giving in. Instead, it came from watching
them learn how to function in ambiguity and get through this
unexpected and abrupt crisis with grit and resilience.

Christina Clancy is the Madison-based author of *The Second Home*
and *Shoulder Season*. Her work has appeared in the *New York Times*,
the *Washington Post*, the *Chicago Tribune*, the *Sun Magazine*, and
elsewhere.

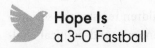

Hope Is
a 3-0 Fastball

LOUIS V. CLARK III

At 3 a.m., I crawl out of bed and deliver the morning newspapers.

At 5:30 a.m., I leave for work.

I work from 6 a.m. until 4 p.m. and arrive home at 4:30 p.m.

After a quick change of clothes, I head up to the baseball diamond, coaching on Monday and Wednesday, umpiring on Tuesday and Thursday. Friday is for Little League practice.

This has been the way of things for close to twenty-five years.

Cue fog and smoke to bring back memories.

The year is 1998. The first-grade neighbor boy, James, has just had a stroke, making it difficult for him to use one arm and one leg. Three years later our youngest son informs us that James is having a tough time growing up. He can't run and jump like the other kids. So we invite him to join our Little League team. We have fifteen players, and each gets to play the same number of innings per game. Everyone gets to pitch at least once during the year.

It's the day of our first Friday practice. God has blessed me with the ability to get just about any nine-to-twelve-year-old to hit the ball where I want. I put James at first base and tell him to stick his glove out. I pitch, like I've been doing for nineteen years, and the batter smacks a ground ball back to the mound. I field the ball, look to first base, then throw as hard as I can to James, who catches it.

Last game of the season arrives. It's the bottom of the last inning, two outs with a runner at second. Walking to the plate is twelve-year-old Preston, the number-one batter in the league.

One of my players yells, "Coach, James didn't get to pitch yet."

I look to his parents, who nod yes.

"Time out!" I call.

50

I motion James to the mound and plop the ball in his palm. The first pitch he throws is "just a little outside," as Harry Doyle would say. His second pitch is short. The third pitch is closer. The count is 3–0, and I'm praying for a fastball down the center. Praying, too, that Preston doesn't hit a line drive and kill my pitcher.

James sets, peers in at the catcher, delivers the pitch. It's a fastball right down the center, followed by a mighty swing as the bottom falls out of the pitch. The bat connects, but just barely—a dribbler to our shortstop.

Field, throw, the ball beats the runner by a mile.

It was James's first win but hardly his last. He went on to play ball throughout high school.

Being quarantined is a good time to reflect on the places where hope hides. But who could have guessed it was hiding in James's 3–0 fastball?

Louis V. Clark III is a poet and storyteller from the Oneida Reservation near Green Bay. After a career of working away from home, he loves being quarantined.

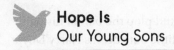

Hope Is
Our Young Sons

CATHRYN COFELL

1.

Because their bodies are a mirror,
because self-reflection captivates,
because they are our heaven,
  even as babies naked and mewling,
  even unfocused, eyes glazed and sleep-crusted,
  even with heads hairless and bite-sized Adam's apples,
because fifteen years from now they'll need allowance, car
  keys, maybe a condom,
because we are the weary queens of upbringing, safety cajolers,
  etiquette breeders,
because women become old news quickly, and hopeless,
because their bodies are a mirror,
because it's easier to let them believe
  in the impossible.

2.

I see the sweet boy from my hip distracted by hope, swaggering
  haughty ripped
squealing hotrod through the suburbs at night cruising for a
  pretty girl hope

pirate hearted manboy heave-hoeing toward the blissful island
  oasis of the know-all
invincible hope

son who will become parent, who grinning and smoothing and
  wide-eyed and whisper
will someday lead me hobbling in the Metamucil

darkness of an assisted-living flat nestled at the edge of his new
   town
happily dying of old age

3.
hope for hot wheels
hope for hot wives
hope for hot politics to cool
and shriveled mamas
to grow old easy
and go down cooing as babies
how much will they suffer
to bathe our bones
how much will they suffer
to rock us to sleep?

Cathryn Cofell is the author of six chapbooks and two full-length poetry collections. In 2020, she received the Christopher Latham Sholes mentoring award from the Council for Wisconsin Writers.

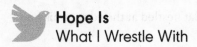

Hope Is
What I Wrestle With

ALEA CROSS

Typical nights, I burn tea lights before bed. I won't admit that I'm scared of the dark; I just have an uneased spirit about darkness. But in bed, I lie with covers wildly situated over me, staring up at the ceiling, allowing the light to pierce the dark. I purse lips, whispering my prayers: "If I should die before I wake, I pray, my lord, my soul you keep."

Typical mornings, I naturally awake, there's trap music that gets progressively louder as I finally tap the alarm clock "snooze" before rolling over, stretching my spine, and tumbling out of bed. This morning isn't like others when I get a text that makes my blush cheeks pale: "uniformed bodies shot her in her sleep."

Typical afternoons, I annoy my teenager until he walks with me. I mean, it is a pandemic-apocalypse; so, between the face guards, close-toed shoes, access-ready hand sanitizer, we brave the fresh air affording more scenery to our lives than 1,067 square feet of quarantine. We speak in tangents as we zigzag across streets avoiding walkers, I mean humans, while being present in the simple pleasures of life. We feel the sun radiate and crisp our melanin. We hear, between laughs, funky Converse and elite Air Jordans crunch branches and hop cracks. I never think I'm unsafe in my neighborhood, maybe surveilled.

I'm not used to virtual run/walks memorializing Black bodies. What happens when someone's white gaze becomes your anxiety. I'm not used to phone calls saying, "They shot him. He was just jogging!"

Typical nights, I lay on the floor sometimes making carpet angels. My favorite yoga position is the Savasana. I breathe deeply, counting down, to release the day's trouble for the day's value. I feel every part of my body awaken with oxygen flowing: *I am alive. I am here. I am in my body.*

I'm not used to masculine wails over the phone: "They did not let him breathe. He cried for his mama in the streets. . . . He still called the officer 'sir' as life escaped his body!"

How am I supposed to stay calm when my chances of dying are exponentially high? The choice is not quite mine: do I die from a virus I can't see, or by the racism I do see? Both are pandemic-genocide to Black bodies!

Where can I find hope for me?
Where can I find hope for my boy?
Where can I find hope for commUNITY?
Where can I find hope for a movement?

I think before I pen:
You need Malcolm to secure Martin.
You need Carson to critique Du Bois and reimagine Douglass
You need Dick Gregory to interpret Farrakhan
You need Sam to sing Ali
You need commUNITY to influence individualism
You need 381 days to catalyze one weekend
You need power in your movement
You need economics to dismantle
You need policy for language
You need sankofa to understand
You need Kasserian Ingera to be present
You need discomfort to feel

Because I hope

To breathe
To sleep and relax in the comforts of my own home
To bird-watch unbothered
To sit in Starbucks and converse
To play my ratchet music
To read a book in my car

To jog
To feel dignity as I ascribe being human

NO MATTER HOW MELANATED MY SKIN IS

Alea Cross is the advising manager at Milwaukee Area Technical College. She is known within her academic community for conversations around race, class, gender, and ableism.

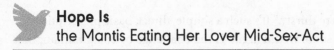

Hope Is
the Mantis Eating Her Lover Mid-Sex-Act

NICK DEMSKE

So there's this quote attributed to Jesus in one of the gnostic gospels, the Gospel of Mary (Magdalene). The quote, in the translation I've read, is, "Be encouraged in the presence of the diversity of forms of nature." The first time I read it, I couldn't make any sense of it, partially because it's wordy. But it's also confusing in context. It comes at the end of a few-sentence answer to the disciple Peter when he asks about sin ("What is the sin of the world?"). So this is ostensibly Jesus's recommendation for safeguarding against discouragement and sin.

That's weird. That's freaking weird. If someone was like, "How do I stop from sinning?" (granted that's not the question here, necessarily), and I was like, "Be encouraged in the presence of the diversity of forms of nature," you'd be like, "Cool, cool . . . Nick is doing drugs."

But isn't that the answer the scientific research keeps confirming for us? I love how ancient wisdom cultures keep getting cosigned by scientific research, millennia after the fact. Science is like, "Turns out meditation is crazy good for you," and gnostic traditions are like, "No shit, y'all. We been said that."

I recently heard second-hand from a woman who does literacy work (like myself) about a study she read that claimed writing about trauma had significantly stronger recovery metrics for vets with PTSD than talking with other vets in group settings. She mentioned this because she was part of a group that helped facilitate such a program. She then off-handedly mentioned that the study also said simply being in nature had significantly better metrics than writing about trauma. So . . . there's that.

This Jesus quote has become a protection mantra for me. "Be encouraged in the presence of the diversity of forms of nature." It's nonsense, at first, but it's basically like saying, "Drink water if you're thirsty." It's such a simple, direct, basic prescription for what some would argue is the challenge of being human, that my impulse is to dismiss it as a mistranslation or something.

But when I turn to the diversity of nature—not by thinking about it or watching it on TV, but being in its presence—it's so utterly insane that it actually arrests everything I think I know about everything and forces me into a childlike state of mind. If I'm feeling hopeless, that sort of just vanishes 'cause what the hell do I know? Scientists estimate that two-thirds of marine life isn't yet discovered. There's exponentially more microorganisms in a single fistful of compost than there are humans beings on this planet. Everything alive shares some amount of DNA, which means we're literally all related. *Damn.*

These are my siblings. These are my parents. My elders and my ancestors. I am them, and they are me. And we are the interconnected web of life. Ain't no climate change, or nuclear war, or shelter in place gonna change that. And I can't help but be swollen with hope at the thought of my big-ass family.

Nick Demske is a poet in Racine, where he also serves as a county supervisor. In his community, he's very involved in local politics, racial justice work, and criminal justice reform.

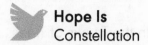

Hope Is
Constellation

BRUCE DETHLEFSEN

one leaf is not a tree
one feather not a wing
no crown a king nor single
note a melody

from darkness are we made
and born alone   our light
our lonely stars though bright
and strong will quickly fade

unless we string the stars
together   choose illumination
then in constellation hope is ours

bring on another day
sing light in common song
shine for the night is long
and dawn is far away

shine for the night is long
and dawn is far away

Bruce Dethlefsen, Wisconsin poet laureate from 2011 to 2012, volunteers writing poems with prisoners and is a member of the Prairie Sands Band. He lives in Westfield, Wisconsin.

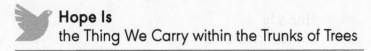

Hope Is
the Thing We Carry within the Trunks of Trees

CONNOR DREXLER

After this is over,
all roads will just be waking
from their first slumber.

Worn bar stools, cafe chairs, picnic benches
thinking they'd had their last chance
at kissing us with splinters, will rise gratefully up
to embrace our prodigal legs.

Down the trail where grass
has finally outgrown our walking, I'll meet you
at the oldest wood available.

The long before long after kind of trees.
The souls so wise I couldn't know
where to start with giving them names
or asking questions worth their wisdom.

When you meet me there, beneath
emerald leaves of another noisy summer,
we'll be reminded our best chance at peace

was to simply outlive our next terror.
To persistently take back
the breath that escapes us.

And what's a greater joy than knowing
to survive any time at all is to win day after day
against powers as big as stars
or too small to see?

Perhaps only
that what often comes with the willingness
to stand tall and rooted

despite what seeks to break us over,
is the ancient mischief of turning
in the same direction

any indomitable hand attempts
to plunge us towards oblivion.
Threatening in each fresh moment

to take to that sky whether or not we
had wings. Whether or
not we had permission to
wield a magic this brave.

Connor Drexler lives in Madison, where he works in the mortgage department of UW Credit Union. His work has been featured in *Black Horse Review*, *Dovecote Magazine*, and *Sky Island Journal*, among others.

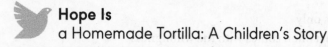

Hope Is
a Homemade Tortilla: A Children's Story

ARACELI ESPARZA

She gets the flour,
She gets the flour and the salt,
She gets the flour, the salt, and the water.
Hungry for my cloud tortillas.
Waiting feels like a year.
The water, the flour, and the salt in a bowl, she begins.
Hungry, Hunger rumbles in my tummy.
She folds in the parts of my cloud and tells the dough how
    much I will love what it will become.
Pitter Patter, thump thun, everyone comes down the stairs and
    now we all squeeze in to watch. Josita, Tommy, Lupita, and
    even little Juanito!
On the table.
She rolls the little ball of masa.
Will I get my own?
Then she centers the masa ball on the tortilla press, pulls the
    lid down, and presses hard.
Pat, pat with her manos!
Five kids watching, waiting, will I get my own?
Smack on the comal on the stove.
"Dale vuelta, Tia! Give it a turn, Tia!" We all whisper shout.
Little Juanito begins to whine, my cloud tortilla dream begins
    to evaporate.
Couple of turns and browning,
Bubbles form, will they Burn?
My cloud tortilla was done all fluffy light and warm.
Tia asks who wants the first tortilla.
Everyone answers, "Me, me, me, me!"
But I say, "Yo por favor!"

Tia gives me the puffy treat I've been waiting for and I float to
the ceiling.

I spread a butter Moon on top of my tortilla, but I see Little
Juanito and I roll it up,

And I give it to him, and I show him how the Cloud Eating is
done.

Araceli Esparza is a poet, writer, and teacher based in Madison. She is
an MFA graduate from Hamline University, with strong migrant farmer
roots, and was named 2015 Women to Watch by *Brava Magazine*.

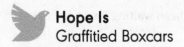

Hope Is
Graffitied Boxcars

JENNIFER FANDEL

Hope is graffitied boxcars
thrumming on the tracks at the crossing
where you stand waiting
while a hot breeze flattens the weeds
and the spice of creosote rises

hope is the palimpsest of messages
that pass before you in pillowy letters
and take you a thousand miles away
to the metallic rattle of the spray can
as the night writer shakes it, trusting
there's a reader out there,
a feeling that might as well be prayer

hope is the crossing arm lifting
and you glimpse what lies on the other side
and you move forward, grounded
by the sound of gravel beneath your feet

Jennifer Fandel teaches poetry classes at the Oakhill Prison and writing classes through University of Wisconsin–Madison Continuing Education. She has also taught writing classes in women's shelters, parks and recreation programs, and grade schools.

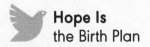
Hope Is
the Birth Plan

STEPHANIE FARRAR

Last year about this time, in the three weeks leading up to my daughter's birth, I spent a lot of time upside down.

The point was to turn the tide of the sea inside and flip this breach baby. I did so, again and again.

I was also having contractions every three to four minutes for three weeks: All I could do was take very short walks, sit, and stand on my head. I knew from my previous experience I had a good chance of having life-threatening complications that endangered both me and the baby, and I had spent a lot of time thinking about this. Because of my experience, because of my research, I had a stark birth plan: "Everybody lives." Nobody wants to hear a pregnant woman talk like this. Nobody is supposed to admit they might die, someday, or possibly soon.

It is so impolite to talk about death, so crass to talk about illness. Nobody is supposed to glimpse mortality as a fact. But this year, all any of us can do is take short walks, sit, and hold the world upside down, patiently for a few weeks.

So, hold it. Hold it, upside down, to turn this tide. Hold this blue pulsing world upside down in your hands because the best birth plan for the new world we will make is just this: "Everybody lives."

Stephanie Farrar is a writer and professor at the University of Wisconsin-Eau Claire, where she teaches and studies American literature. She is the coeditor of *Dickinson In Her Own Time*.

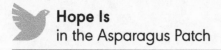

Hope Is
in the Asparagus Patch

CHRIS FINK

Each day this spring finds me kneeling at the edge of the new asparagus patch, looking for shoots. The tiny purple spears don't erupt messily from the soil like a bean sprout does, but emerge rather stealthily, almost mystically. I check the patch first thing in the morning, dress the two new purple shoots in compost, then come back an hour later and find two more. Sometimes they seem to arrive even as I'm staring, and I think this is a miracle. It's really true. My own asparagus patch.

The asparagus of my youth was a wild and rare delectable, its feathery fronds woven with family mythology. In those days, my dad kept a vegetable garden, but the asparagus he brought to the table was bootleg. A locomotive engineer for the Milwaukee Road, he was known to halt a whole line of freight when he spotted asparagus along the tracks. He drove the family to distraction on springtime car trips to the Kettle Moraine, taking the Buick through the curves achingly slowly, his eye on the ditches.

Quarantined this April, my eye wandered to my own vegetable garden. Too soon. When the state began to open up, I sneaked out to the greenhouse for garden seeds. There at the end cap of the checkout, looking like great gray arachnids, asparagus crowns sunned themselves in a messy heap, beckoning from long ago. If not this spring, rooted to this patch of earth, then when? I bought two bundles, a Jersey Knight and a Purple Passion.

When I borrowed my friend Mike's tiller, I'm sure he could already envision the pitiful first draft of my asparagus patch. I tend to jump into projects. I read directions only after I'm in the middle of something and find myself stumped. "Take your time," he said. "Plant it like it will be there forever." So, after I tilled a skinny stretch of weeds, I cracked open the pamphlet that came with the tangle of crowns. What was all this about compost tea, wood ash, and a measuring tape? Does a ditch plant that volunteers among the spiderwort need such pampering? Then I counted the crowns. Forty-nine! One for each year of my life. Oh, my. Had the greenhouse shorted me one just to plant the seed of kismet? I gulped. My tilled row could fit maybe ten.

So, with Mike's good counsel in mind, I bent once more to the tiller. I would put the time in now and then reap year after year of bounty, right there at the edge of the yard. No locomotive required. I'll just wander out barefoot with a kitchen knife. But I'll have to wait. Asparagus takes three years to fulfill its promise. What will the world be like in three years? So far, by my count, thirty-eight of the forty-nine stalks have emerged. Taming wild asparagus is all very painstaking, if you want to do it right. I'm still not sure that I have.

Chris Fink is a professor of English and environmental studies at Beloit College, where he edits the *Beloit Fiction Journal*. His book of short fiction, *Add This to the List of Things That You Are*, won a 2020 Society of Midland Authors fiction prize.

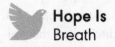 **Hope Is**
Breath

SUSAN FIRER

8 Minutes and 46 Seconds

My Catholic father knelt next to his bed
each night. He rested his praying hands
on top of his mattress. His hands
shaped the same architecture as my
morning hands now make in Anjali Mudra.
Until she no longer could, my mother knelt
in her summer dress, in her summer
garden, planting yellow and orange
chrysanthemums. Knees are meant
to kneel. The nuns in Catholic school
taught me how to genuflect, a quick one-knee kneel.
Colin Kaepernick taught me the strength
in kneeling. So far worldwide 900,000
people have died in the COVID-19 pandemic.
Unaccountable numbers have died in the
"pandemic within the pandemic." People
across the world are out in upended streets,
protesting the cop's knee on George Floyd's
neck, the knee that crushed Floyd's beautiful
face into the street, that crushed all life's breath
from him. Across the world in Australia,
in Boston, Chicago, in Denver, England,
France, Germany, in Hollywood, India,
Japan, Kenya, London, in Milwaukee,
New York, Philadelphia, Quebec,
in Sweden, Texas, Utah, Virginia,
Washington, DC, and Zimbabwe
people are honoring George Floyd.

A planetary throng of voices shouts
"I can't breathe,"
"Say his name,"
"No Justice, no Peace."
The chants challenging
violences and silences.
To kneel is a spiritual act.
To breathe is a spiritual act.
People are kneeling.
I am relearning how to kneel.
Knees are meant to kneel.
In prayer, in protest, in yoga, in gardens,
in love, in respect, in burning cities,
people are kneeling.

Susan Firer is the author of six full-length books of poetry, most recently *The Transit of Venus*. From 2008 to 2010, she was Milwaukee poet laureate. In 2015, Firer was awarded a NEA Fellowship in Poetry.

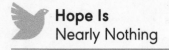

Hope Is
Nearly Nothing

MAX GARLAND

I love Emily Dickinson's famous poem on hope, but this morning, it's her contemporary, Walt Whitman, who comes to mind. I "bequeath myself to the dirt," he said. "Look for me under your boot soles," he said. I'm holding Walt to his words. "Keep encouraged," he said. "Missing me one place, search another."

This morning I'm searching another, and another after that. A cold gray sky hovers over this late March day, and our portion of the planet here in the Chippewa Valley is snow covered again. Snow raggedly outlines the otherwise bare trees and grants the evergreens a frosted look, a sort of senior moment, you might say.

I'm remembering what composes a snowflake. I mean, what's at the crux of the crystal hexagon? Before it can form, briefly float, inevitably fall to outline, and lightly weigh upon the branches? Before it can clot the treads of tires, whitecap the neighborhood houses?

It's just dirt, of course, that forms the nucleus, the cold heart of snow. A fleck of dust, speck of grit, maybe a discarded and upswept pollen grain. It takes nearly nothing, in fact, but *nearly nothing* is vastly different from *nothing*. It's that cast-off floating particle of grit in the upper air that allows molecules of ice to be true to their hexagonal blueprint, branch, and elaborate into the various shapes of snowflakes—lattice, lace, diamond dust, aggregate, column, needle, or my personal favorite—the stellar dendrite.

In this season of viral distancing, quarantine, and genuine suffering, here, this morning, the fourth week of March (I'm going out on a limb here) comes the small gift of spring snow. I think of how something so tiny, *nearly nothing*, dust or pollen, is seized by the frigid upper air, then branches into performance mode, a kind of beatification of grit, that falls and now covers what I can see of my town from the window of my own isolation.

My hope on this crisis-ridden morning is the audacity of grit, those castaway particles of nearly nothing that allow the crystalline pattern of ice to launch into beauty, cold beauty, sure, but the point is that the smallest thing—dirt, dust, grit—seeds the miraculous, both outside of us, and inside.

I admire the acts of obvious heroism (doctors, nurses, emergency workers), but this snowy morning, it's also the grit of the girl stocking grocery shelves, the trucker, baker, convenience store clerk, ordinary neighbors keeping the human grid alive—repairing furnaces, feeding and dressing our quarantined elders who once did the same for us—that's hope for me. That's the human manifestation of the unspectacular grit at the heart of the snowflake.

"I depart as air," Walt Whitman said. "I shake my white locks at the runaway sun," he said. "Keep encouraged," he said. I'm trying, Walt, remembering that it's also words—empathetic, heartfelt, trivial, humorous, distracting; it's the irrepressible grit *of* humanity at the core of our impulse to speak, write, sing, listen, to bridge the distance with words—that constitutes hope for me, and keeps me encouraged.

Max Garland's most recent book is *The Word We Used for It*, winner of the Brittingham Poetry Prize. A former rural mail carrier and first-generation college student, Garland is professor emeritus at the University of Wisconsin-Eau Claire and a former poet laureate of Wisconsin.

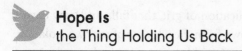

Hope Is
the Thing Holding Us Back

JAY GILBERTSON

Think how little hope has accomplished. We hope for this to happen, hope for that to go away, hope for the best. But when we look beneath that romantic wish and see it clearly for what it is—a puff of maybe, a twinkling of tomorrow, a dash of next week, month, year. A place where doubt, then fear, can slip in, take over. Then hope does what it always does, always will.

Hope dies.

Hope has no place in this new era. This idyllic word packed full of good intentions, sealed with a promise, is what has long prevented us from doing the work, and being our best, and setting ourselves free.

In this new place we are in, it's time to set hope free.

Stand tall, breathe in what matters;

Black Lives Matter.

COVID is not a hoax.

Words have power.

I have known hope. We used to be friends. Growing up gay, hoping someone would see me, hoping AIDS away, hoping to marry who I loved, hoping for equality.

Hope never came.

Change did.

Hope is the thing holding us back. Action is the path forward. We can no longer hope for change to come or hope for someone else to be the change.

We, you and me, we are the change we have been waiting for, the change we have been dying for, the change already happening.

Next time you hope for this or hope for that—don't.
Instead, be the change.
We are the change we have been waiting for—the wait is over.

Jay Gilbertson lives in Prairie Farm, Wisconsin. He is a published author, husband, and pumpkin seed oil farmer, and he believes in you.

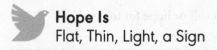

Hope Is
Flat, Thin, Light, a Sign

SUSAN GLOSS

Hope is flat.

Hope is a friend on a bicycle beneath bare locust branches and graphite skies. She leaves a sourdough starter on my porch, rings the bell, and pedals away. This friendly game of ding-dong ditch would be odd in other times. Nothing is normal, though. Not now. That afternoon, in a corner of the kitchen, I begin a cycle of weighing and waiting, feeding and fermenting, that will give structure to the uncertain days ahead. My first attempt at bread falls flat. I end up with a passable pizza dough instead of a boule. With repetition, though, I start to see results. I become someone who stocks bread flour in the pantry. Apparently, I am not alone. The supermarket tacks up a sign in the baking aisle: "One bag of flour per family, per day." I buy a five-pound bag. It's gone in two weeks.

Hope is thin.

Hope is a packet of snap pea seeds, purchased at the corner hardware store just before it closed its doors and restricted its business to "curbside pickup only"—a new phrase that becomes part of the popular lexicon, like "flatten the curve" and "social distancing." My sons and I spend an afternoon tucking seeds into dirt in black plastic trays. Each day, they take turns with a spray bottle, soaking the soil and sometimes each other. They lose interest after a week or so without visible results, so I take over the watering. I don't mind. Unlike the kids and the dog, who remind me a thousand times a day that they are hungry, the seeds say nothing while they wait for nourishment. From their silence, sprouts emerge, thin and tenacious.

Hope is light.

Hope is a gallon of paint. It's the feeling that, if I can't control what's happening outside the walls of my home—the sickness and the death and the fear—then I can at least control what's on my walls. I have an overpowering desire for everything to be lighter, brighter. I need contrast to combat so much heaviness.

Hope is a sign.

Hope is a homemade sign in the window. It's a rainbow the kids and I colored for neighbors to see while walking by. It's a "thank you" spelled out for frontline workers who deliver groceries and mail and takeout from our favorite restaurants, which we pray can hold on.

Later, at the tail end of spring, just as the pink peonies in the side yard are blooming, we make another sign as our country mourns the killing of George Floyd: BLACK LIVES MATTER.

We should have made this sign months ago, years ago. Floyd is not the first unarmed Black American killed by a police officer. Not nearly. We should have made a sign for all of them—each life, each death—but yet we did not. And so, this sign is for all of them. We know it is too late. But still we hope it is not too late.

Susan Gloss is the best-selling author of two novels and the recipient of a Wisconsin Library Association Outstanding Achievement Award. She lives in Madison with her family.

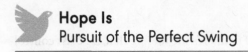

Hope Is
Pursuit of the Perfect Swing

NEAL GRIFFIN

Imagine the misery of a fifteen-year-old denied the joy of high school baseball. A long-anticipated freshman season swept aside by a microscopic opponent. But it's not just about baseball. It's about being in a classroom, not a Zoom room. Hanging out with friends, sitting shoulder to shoulder at lunch. Making weekend plans to see a movie, where the long wait jostling in line is half the fun. For teenagers living through the pandemic of 2020, everyday life has become a disheartening list of social deprivations.

So how hard should a dad be on a boy who begins to withdraw? Who spends so much time on the couch it's like he was poured there? Then again, maybe instead of going all judge and jury on the kid, the best thing a dad can do is help him find hope.

"What say we go outside?" I extend the offer of a baseball bat. "Work on your swing a bit? You're gonna need it next spring."

I resist reacting to his sullen stare accompanied by an off-putting shrug. Don't judge him, I remind myself. Help him find hope.

"Come on. Corona won't last forever." I coax him to a standing position and push him toward the door. "You wanna be ready, right?"

Outside the sun dominates a crisp Wisconsin April sky, tailor-made for baseball. A pair of swans trumpet a greeting from a nearby lake. Towering birch trees in full bud sway in the breeze, taking on the part of anxious spectators. Unable to resist, he snatches the lumber from my hand. He rolls his shoulders and twists the bat in his grip, arms straight out, staring at the familiar barrel, proud of its many blemishes. He waves it menacingly, then gives it a cocky spin above his head. I tee up a ball and in that moment the crush of COVID-19 is set aside. I see a glimmer of hope.

"Go easy," I say. "It's been a while."

Sure enough, he tops the first one and the ball takes a rusty dribble into the net. I feel the stir of my own optimism when, without hesitation, he tees up another. This time the connection is rock solid but not yet full power. Then, he begins to bring it.

Before the first bucket is empty, the baseballs are coming off the tee like bullets shot from a gun, smacking the bullseye of the net. Each swing grows stronger. Head down. Palms up. The torque of his hips fully engaged. After fifty cuts, I turn the tee to the woods a few hundred feet away.

"Let 'er rip."

He adjusts the height, imagining a delivery he'd make any pitcher live to regret. The swing is pure, the ball clears the trees and, in his mind, sails deep into a cheering crowd.

Slowly it returns. The swagger of an athlete. The resilience of youth. A boy in pursuit of the perfect swing, finding hope for all his seasons yet to come.

Neal Griffin grew up in Eau Claire, a diehard fan of Yount, Thomas, Coop, and all the other Wallbangers of the bittersweet '82 season. These days Neal, his wife, and their family have a home in Burnett County.

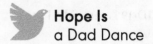

Hope Is
a Dad Dance

MATTHEW GUENETTE

I was scrambling eggs for the kids
but I wanted something more, something epic like to take
the moon in my hands. What other powers do I have?
The kids, captive at home for at least
the next month, how to protect them when even the jungle
gyms are canceled and every cough inspires a nightmare.
What else should we do, send them out in hazmat suits
with their safety scissors? Vote? Haven't we tried
all that? There's a feeling I want to get us back to,
like when I was thirteen and it hardly mattered
if Gorbachev and Reagan waved their intercontinental
pricks at each other, it was all the same
and nothing a game of H-O-R-S-E or *Purple Rain*
couldn't fix. I had one job, I plated the eggs
and thought of us climbing back into the trees
to hurl water balloons at the suckers who think
they know better. That's when I knew better, when I knew
I had another job. I hiked up my boxers like a thonged
superhero. The kids in the next room waiting at
the table: Are the eggs almost done? You have no idea,
I said. Hold tight! Then I tied on my little cape
of sunlight and danced their way.

Matthew Guenette is the author of three full-length poetry collections, *Vasectomania*, *American Busboy*, and *Sudden Anthem*. He teaches composition and creative writing at Madison College and lives on the east side with his wife, their two children, and a 20-pound cat named Butternut.

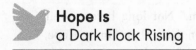

Hope Is
a Dark Flock Rising

NICHOLAS GULIG

In Dickinson's *314*, the poet turns her hope into a
bird. I'm almost 40. Because they've started coming
back, I imagine this desire blurs into a horned lark.
It's February, cold, and local outlets announce the
presence of the virus in Wisconsin. Such is the power
of metaphor. According to reports, the patient walked
alone into a hospital. My body slows into its history.
In periods of lasting isolation, the theory of allopatric
speciation contends that over time some birds
phenotypically respond to their geography. "How
are you doing?" my daughter writes in a letter to her
friend. Metaphors conflate. Separating species, this
variance in habitat demands a new vocabulary. "Their
symptoms were consistent." In the open field between
an object and its import, language clutches at the air.
"I really hate this virus." And yet, for Dickinson, the
bird that hope becomes is either prior to, or after
speech. "A thing with feathers that perches in the
soul." These symptoms include recurrent coughing,
fever, and fatigue. An endless, inner singing. Often,
the body aches and does so deeply, a pain that lasts
for days and echoes in the muscle, in the bone. At
first, I paid no mind. If birds of the same type are kept
apart for long enough, they cease to see themselves
in others of their kind, their common song no longer
a reunion. In some cases, the lips and face turn blue
from lack of oxygen. The song moves in and out of us.
Spreading exponentially. In a post-pandemic world,
the exchange between a symbol and its referent now
requires the strange catastrophe of breath, what

Dickinson calls "a storm." Not long before their fever, the patient had been to see their family. Hope, it seems, cannot be parted from the maelstrom. My first thought, if I remember, was not a thought at all. I heard it "in the chillest land—and on the strangest sea." A blue silence rose within me. Every day, at three o'clock precisely, the girls in my neighborhood stand alone in separate driveways and yell each other's names across the boulevard. My faith in art is that the bird exists as an insistence and can and will disrupt the context of its singing, its small voice passing through an air we now imagine poisoned. Crossing continents and oceans, one presumes the patient had wanted to see the faces of their loved ones. To be a form held tight against another. I, too, desire to be a form held tight against another. Every night I grab a beer from my refrigerator and talk nostalgic with my friends. The virus is a line of air connecting us to people we'll never meet, whose names occur in languages we'll never speak, dark tongues. "The Department of Human Services is operating with an abundance of caution." We are older now, and lonely. The existence of extrinsic barriers obstructs the call-like variance of our transmissions. It is difficult to think of hope in Dickinson's work without remembering that when I read it, I find myself beside myself, unspooled in a different wilderness. As if for the first time, we are learning how to see each other, our faces glitched and framed by our computers. Often, her language falls apart, the frequent dashes suturing the starts and stops of fragments, a kind of calling out from deep within the terror of a pause. "The patient is being monitored." In moments of extremity, the song arrives as if the storm had beckoned it. "Dear Cubby, I wish that we could play." Here, where no one is themselves, we're telling the story over, night by night. The first death, then the second. Our language hangs in air. The friend my daughter writes to is the daughter of a man I've known since we were children, so when they set their letters in the mailbox, it feels like we do too, our history returning across the landscape, a time and place no longer present moving through our kids. All of us are breathing. The structure of our lungs expands to house the living remnants. My daughter stares beyond the window. There, in Wisconsin, the first returning migratory birds perch on the snow-bright stalks of goldenrod. Sheltered though we are, our hope is that in which we speak to stitch ourselves together. Dickinson was wrong; this requires everything. "The patient is now at home." Months before the spring, the horned larks gather in dark flocks, picking through the ice and stubble, searching for hidden seeds. This is their geography. When frightened, the flock alights as one, a single entity twisting swiftly, their lisping callnotes disappearing in the half-imagined distance of their song.

Nicholas Gulig is a Thai-American poet from Wisconsin. Educated in Montana, Iowa, and Colorado, Gulig earned a Fulbright Fellowship to Bangkok, Thailand, in 2011. He lives in Fort Atkinson and teaches at the University of Wisconsin–Whitewater.

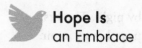

Hope Is
an Embrace

KATY HACKWORTHY

Hope is an embrace

which I'm learning takes many forms: the elderly couple
eating sandwiches over a kitchen sink, their love
encyclopedically etched into sagging faces, or the teens
tangled under a sizable spruce across the street, their tenderness
so delicate I have to look away, or the child
forcing his face into the cat's fur, inviting the rough ritual
of a tongue traveling across his forehead, their bond
becoming a promise.

We are all learning new methods of enveloping each other
without the tools of touch—we share poems in place
of firm squeezes, palm in palm, across the dinner table.
Instead of arms slung swiftly across shoulders, we share songs
to remedy all the ways we don't know how to say "I love you."
Our eyes entangle and instead of cradling a cheek
in cupped hands, or brushing loose locks behind an ear,
we honor this new way of holding each other the best we can,
refusing to look away.

Katy Hackworthy is an organizer, caregiver, and writer. She lives in South
Minneapolis with her cat, Long Walt, but her heart will always reside in
the woods of northern Wisconsin.

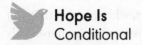

Hope Is
Conditional

DAVID HADBAWNIK

Maybe all we really have is what's right in front of us. So many of the plans that we made, dreams we had for the future—even something so ordinary as an upcoming ballgame, birthday party, or vacation—has been taken away by the COVID crisis. At times it feels like we are all, each of us in our little self-isolated circles, standing on a tiny island watching the water rise, swallowing things one by one.

Last year at this time my wife and I, and our soon-to-be one-year-old son, were living in Kuwait. Tina and I had full-time jobs as professors at an all-English private university. We were making good money, and we enjoyed our work and our colleagues. But our tolerance for life in Kuwait, with its harsh weather and social restrictions, had run its course, especially with an active son who wants to play outside. So I reluctantly waded into the job market once again.

I was delighted when a late-breaking opportunity arose as a visiting assistant professor in the English Department at Wisconsin–Eau Claire. Two great friends of ours from grad school days were professors there, and we'd heard good things about the school and the area. Luckily—in a lightning-fast interview, job offer, and moving process that is a whole different story—things worked out, and we arrived in Eau Claire in August 2019. Our friends helped a lot, and we found the city itself and my new colleagues to be incredibly welcoming as well. The ability to walk outside in the pleasant summer air, visit the farmers market, go running on trails along the river—this was a miracle, one we didn't take for granted after four years in the desert.

But I couldn't relax for long. A position as visiting assistant professor is transitional and transactional—you are providing temporary, needed labor to a university, with the idea that you leverage it into something more permanent elsewhere. This is the nature of the beast in today's precarious state of higher education.

Thus, I continued applying for jobs. Through an agency, I was referred for a job as "head of academics" at a small, private, Muslim-centered K–12 school in Austin, Texas. I eagerly applied and was soon invited to interview. This seemed like an unbelievable opportunity. My wife and I had met in San Marcos, just south of Austin, and we still had many friends in the area. After ten-plus interviews, both over the phone and in person on a campus visit, I was offered the job in early February. I negotiated and signed a five-year contract soon after, and with relief and joy we began telling friends and family about our impending move.

And then came COVID.

Looking back now, it's easy to see the warning signs. The early rumblings from China, the growing alarm in the rest of the world, the (false) reassurances from the Trump administration that we wouldn't have to worry about an epidemic here. As recently as the second week of March, I was still planning to fly to Austin over our spring break to observe some classes at the school, still planning to meet with real estate agents to find out what kind of housing our stretched budget could afford, still gleefully making plans with our Austin friends.

In the space of just a few days in mid-March, everything changed. Austin's famous SXSW festival was canceled (along with the NBA season, Coachella, and many other events). Suddenly it became obvious I couldn't fly to Austin anytime soon. Then I received an ominous e-mail from my contact at the school, telling me they'd already had parents unable to pay tuition and were worried about enrollment for next year. Soon after that I spoke with the school owner, and she asked me to give her until mid-April to try to figure things out.

I said yes—what else could I say?—and waited with chagrin as the virus ravaged New York, California, most of the country, while millions of people were instantly out of work. We began letting friends and family know that we might not be moving to Austin after all. And I informed my (very understanding) department chair that I might need to rescind my resignation.

A few days ago, I received a regretful message from the school that, indeed, they would not be able to honor my contract. Though we'd come to expect such news, it was still a blow. It still is a blow. In just a few weeks we'd gone from dreaming of buying a house and enjoying the type of security that would see us toward retirement to wondering how long we could afford our current rent, and what kind of employment prospects might lie ahead in this dark new world.

Is there hope? I refuse to subscribe to wild-eyed optimism—the wishful thinking of an administration that until recently claimed the virus would simply disappear in warmer weather—even as I refuse to submit to despair. COVID has already taken so much from so many of us. Twenty thousand dead and counting at the time of this writing. Millions unemployed. Frontline workers and caregivers still without basic protections. And the small, personal things the rising tide takes away: the party we'd been planning for our son's second birthday, and Tina's brother flying in from Europe to celebrate with us.

What we're left with is what's right in front of us. The still-miraculous gift of taking walks outside in nature. My son's face as he smiles and laughs and sings, blessedly oblivious to the worries of the pandemic. These moments give me the spark to get through the otherwise monotonous days. And they fuel my cautious hope, leavened with anger at what's been lost. That hope is conditional on turning the anger into action to transform the world we go back to. A world in which we no longer tolerate the systemic inequalities, and the underfunded and overwhelmed health-care system, that have made this crisis so much worse. A world in which we prepare for such storms rather than waiting for them to sweep over us.

David Hadbawnik is a poet, translator, and medieval scholar. His translation *Aeneid: Books 1–6* was published by Shearsman Books in 2015. He is currently visiting assistant professor of writing at University of Wisconsin–Eau Claire.

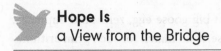

Hope Is
a View from the Bridge

JOHN HILDEBRAND

Dogs are the chief beneficiaries of shelter-in-place in my neighborhood. They give us license to move about and expect, in return, longer walks and more of them. So instead of turning around at the river and heading home, my black lab and I cross the bridge to the other side, a pleasant walk now that the streets are empty.

One bright morning as we were crossing the bridge, a voice boomed behind us, "I am the ALPHA and the OMEGA! *Whaaaahhoooo!*"

The dog and I picked up our pace.

"I AM the Alpha and the Omega! *Yee-hah!*"

Reluctant to turn around and see what sort of face would match the braying voice, I kept walking. Only after we were safely across the bridge did I turn to look. A young man, his face obscured in a hoodie, was bouncing down the other side of the street on the balls of his feet while shouting into a cell phone, "I AM the Alpha and the Omega! *Whooooo-eeee!*"

Overheard cell phone conversations are often a source of amusement, but for the life of me I couldn't imagine who was on the receiving end of such a monologue—a dealer? A therapist? And I'll never know because the guy in the hoodie disappeared down Water Street.

Well, I thought, that's one way to deal with a deadly pandemic, get so strung out that you're the only reality. Gloomy thoughts of mortality? Not for Mr. Alpha and Omega!

I know the feeling. Lately I cannot face the evening news without pouring a stiff drink to fortify myself against the day's numbers—how many infected, how many hospitalized, how many dead. Sometimes it feels as if you're being stalked by the numbers—as they go up, your personal number goes down, edging ever closer to that big goose egg, zero. And euphoria, drug-induced or otherwise, is no match for such grim arithmetic. For one thing, it wears off.

One of the pleasures of dog walking is being tied to a creature that lives solely in the here and now, and when the black lab finishes his business, we head home. At mid-span on the bridge I'll lean over the railing to see if any fish are holding in the current. Rivers are good places to contemplate time. You look down into the moving water knowing there's a source far upstream in some dark, reedy swamp and, many miles downstream, a yawning mouth, but what you see isn't the beginning or the end but the continuous, unbroken flow of things. Looking at a river, any river, makes me feel hopeful. And hope is the bridge that allows us to cross from the awful now to the better days ahead even if we can't quite see them from here.

John Hildebrand is the author of numerous books, including *Long Way Round*, *Mapping the Farm*, and *The Heart of Things*. He is an emeritus professor at the University of Wisconsin–Eau Claire.

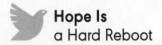

Hope Is
a Hard Reboot

LUONG HUYNH

Dear Valued Customer,

I am sorry to hear that you have been sheltered in your home for the last eighty-eight days. I understand how frustrating this experience must be for you. Please know that we value your time and will be forwarding all concerns to the appropriate departments.

As for your primary issue, rest assured that your country is not defective and that it is simply an older, out-of-production model that, from time to time, will need upgrading to process the heavy data loads of current events.

To alleviate your performance issues, I would highly suggest the following:

- Hard reboot your social contract
- Defrag your most vulnerable communities and populations
- Install an up-to-date public health-care program (detailed instructions can be found at socialsafety.nets)

I appreciate you making us aware of your concerns and please feel free to reach out again if your problems persist.

Sincerely,
Luong Huynh
Customer Service Representative

Luong Huynh lives in Eau Claire and works in disaster response for a national nonprofit. In his time off, Luong is a freelance event photographer and regular contributor to *Volume One*.

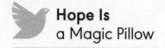

Hope Is
a Magic Pillow

SARAH JAYNE JOHNSON

When I was around ten, I got the stomach flu, and it changed me. For whatever reason, this singular night of porcelain companionship triggered a lifetime of hypochondria and illness-related anxiety that made me feel hopeless, lonely, and stressed. I started changing the way I did things to reflect a little voice in my head telling me if I didn't do things a certain way, I'd get sick. A voice that would circle and spiral until I was crying nearly every night when I went to bed. I wanted so badly to have control over the thing that I feared most, and I started to lose my mind when I couldn't have it.

One night, while wiping big tears from my eyes, my dad came and sat at the foot of my bed. He had brought me his coveted "magic pillow" that made any big, terrible thing melt away from the moment your ear touched the pillowcase.

"Okay, so what's wrong?" he asked.

"I don't know, I just, I don't want to get sick," I said, between shallow, uneven gulps of air.

"Well," my dad said, "that's not always up to you. Sometimes we have to realize that a lot of things in life are out of our control, and that's okay. You can only do all you can do." He then wrapped the covers around me, fluffed my pillow, and my fear subsided a bit.

The world is a giant, beautiful, and scary sphere spinning around whether we like it or not. Now more than ever, it's important to lean on each other (figuratively, of course) to hold this big blue ball in place. Comfort yourself by comforting others. Grieve openly and in unison with those you love. Be vulnerable from afar, and recognize that hopelessness only wins if you let it. Talk to the people you love because, chances are, they're going

to love you right back. And when all of this is over, and we start
to settle back into normalcy, that love will still linger.

So grab your magic pillow. And maybe call your dad. You can
only do all you can do.

Sarah Jayne Johnson grew up in La Crosse. She is a writer and community advocate in Eau Claire.

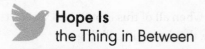

Hope Is
the Thing in Between

KENDALL KARTALY

Growing up in Altoona, Wisconsin, I often felt restless even with its assuring city slogan "A great place to grow." I knew the curves of the street, the potholes, the sun's slant, the bored motions of the checkout boy in aisle five. I knew the frame of the trees, the smell of the pine, the exhale when I rolled into the driveway: home. It was a certain kind of burgeoning push to explore the worlds I have never seen before, often in books, finding refuge and rest.

As a growing teacher in college, what began as a love of Polish poetry turned into teaching English in Poland through a Fulbright grant. Here, I was caught between two worlds: immersing myself in Polish culture, and sharing aspects of American and Wisconsin life. My Polish friends evolved into family, with holiday celebrations, lazy weekends, evening walks, knowing where to put things in the kitchen, door open. Likewise, my students' curiosity found me explaining that one of the oldest Altoona streets is indeed Division Street, describing the way the trees move, the seasons change, the fresh blueberries at Weaver's Country Store in summer, the anticipation of a snow day while watching the television screen, and hiking with my mom.

I cultivated such an appreciation for both of these spaces. I was often caught between the tenses "is" and "was," not due to grammatical uncertainty, but because I could not quite find the tense that fit the feeling. Now, at an international school teaching students of more than thirty different nationalities, I sense some of my students wrestling with this liminality too, especially during this time of uncertainty.

For me, being on a different continent, I am in between the spaces of here and there—home—in Poland and Wisconsin. The dissonance used to be when I was at my favorite *kawiarnia* and people would greet me with *"Cześć"* when the sudden lilts of "Holocene" by Bon Iver played, unexpectedly, as the workers were rearranging *chleb* and *sernik* at the counter. It used to be in the extra pause when I would fill out a form stating "home address." Now it is in the confusion of messages when both Polish and American friends write, "Are you staying here or going back?" "Are you there or here?"

Where exactly is the here and where exactly is the there? I wonder. When do you claim a place as your home?

And now, as I walk in the streets of Warsaw to the Kabaty Forest, I close my eyes toward the sky, like my mom used to tell me, and listen to the trees, like crashing waves, transporting me from here to there. I am reminded that trees can sense one another in between the spaces they give and leave and that is delightfully amazing; perhaps, a reminder that I am rooted halfway around the world and at the same time rolling into the driveway on a quiet Wisconsin street.

Kendall Kartaly was born and raised in Altoona, Wisconsin, and is currently living in Warsaw, Poland. As a writer and English teacher she sees the power of stories, art, and representation helping the world speak and listen, trying to search for and name the "thing" in between it all.

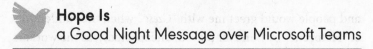

Hope Is
a Good Night Message over Microsoft Teams

EMILY KASSERA

The thoughts my eighth-graders choose to vocalize fascinate me. Sometimes, they're sweet: "You're like the *best* listener." Sometimes they're backhanded: "If you weren't old and if you wore cooler shoes, I would totally want to be your friend." (I'm twenty-three, for reference.) But most of the time, they're contrary: "I don't want to be here."

That one's my favorite. Most students mutter it subconsciously from time to time, but a few really enjoy the way it feels on their tongues. Like an Olympic javelin toss, I can see them preparing to launch those words. I'll be up there, jiving with the lesson, other kids are loving it, I'll start circling the classroom for one-on-one help, and these folks . . . they'll look me dead in the eye when I get to them and let it fall from their lips like it's weightless: *I don't want to be here.*

It used to crush me, but not anymore. How could I let it? They're only saying what we're all thinking. Do I sometimes wish I could stand up in the middle of a stressful meeting and say, "I don't want to be here"? Yes. Do I think it on particularly tough days when I have things outside of school causing me worry? Absolutely. The thing is, "I don't want to be here" is just the blunt way of saying all of the things adults have invented niceties to damper. How could I fault a fourteen-year-old for that?

Right now, however, the global pandemic has quite literally forced us to "not be here." Schools are officially closed for the remainder of the year. While I'm devastated to lose the in-person aspect of my student teaching semester, I couldn't help but let my mind drift to the *I don't want to be here* kids. Were they shocked? Were they elated? Were they toasting sparkling white grape juice and making celebratory TikToks?

I didn't know the answer, but a week after schools closed, I sent all of my students a check-in message. I asked how they were and assured them that I was eager to stay connected through our district's chosen platform, Microsoft Teams. I got several responses later that day with everything from Netflix recommendations, to photos of pets, to recipes for their mom's banana bread.

That was almost one month ago, now—one month since I sent that first check in—but just two nights ago, my phone buzzed on my dresser. It was 10 p.m. I grumbled and rose reluctantly from bed to check it. There was a reply . . . to my one-month-old message, from the poster child of *I don't want to be here*: "goodnight ms kassera. i miss ur class."

As a University of Wisconsin–Eau Claire English and theatre education graduate, **Emily Kassera** now teaches eighth-grade English at Altoona Middle School in Altoona, Wisconsin. She's thrilled to be reading, writing, and making theatre with those hip Chippewa Valley teens.

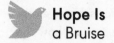

Hope Is
a Bruise

DASHA KELLY HAMILTON

Paintball pellets batter shoulders
and thighs at 190 miles per hour
I count the purplish bruises and
smile at the post vision of us toasting
laughing, being vibrantly alive

The woman who pierced my nose
Rushed outside afterwards for a cigarette
Whether my nostril or her nerves were to blame
We both survived an ordeal that day
I don't think of the sweat on her lip
or the tears on my cheek when my jeweled
Black nose disrupts canonical spaces

Agony delineates child bearing from child rearing
Pain is the anticipated toll: the impossible stretch of skin and
    orifice,
wrenching of organs, the pinch and nip of nursing
I received no pamphlets about the pangs of panic and
    impotence
The deep marrow rupture when their ache explodes beyond
    your reach

A formation of police fired rubber bullets at my child
200 feet per second in defense of hatred and spiteful ignorance
She raged back in protest until her throat rasped, her heels
blistered and she relented into sobs once safe in our home,
    in my arms

They gassed and maced my baby. She marched again the next
   day.
And the next and the next and the next and the next
Hope is a bruise, a nervous smoke and an unrelenting cavalry

Dasha Kelly Hamilton was named Wisconsin poet laureate for 2021 to
2022 and served as Milwaukee poet laureate from 2019 to 2021. She is a
writer, performance artist, and creative change agent, applying the creative process to facilitate dialogues around human and social wellness.

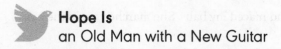

Hope Is
an Old Man with a New Guitar

DION KEMPTHORNE

In his book *Until the End of Time*, Brian Greene, a physicist searching for meaning in a mechanical universe, quotes Yip Harburg, the author of "Over the Rainbow" (voted best song of the twentieth century), as follows: "Words make you think a thought. Music makes you feel a feeling. But a song makes you feel a thought." Then Greene writes: "*Feel a thought.* For me, that captures the essence of artistic truth."

For me, too. And perhaps for Emily, whose "thing with feathers" is about song, the bird's in music and hers in words. And just this morning cardinals were singing the first two notes of Stephen Foster's refrain in "Hard Times Come Again No More." *Hard times, hard times,* they whistled over and over. But what to think or feel or sing about the calamity of COVID-19?

Mourning takes so many forms.

By sheer coincidence, last fall I decided to take guitar lessons. Here's what I found at the very start of Hal Leonard's *Guitar Method* for beginners: Beethoven's "Ode to Joy." Five notes on strings one and two, which, like a cardinal, I played over and over. And what an added joy, when asked what I liked to play, to be able to say, well, mainly Beethoven. Now, this spring, after joining a Zoom guitar class and having safer-at-home practice time, I'm playing better than I ever thought I could.

And what a comfort it's been to have a guitar to self-isolate with. It's soothing to hold and hear, to sound out, by hand and heart, in warm tones of rosewood and cedar, harmonies of life and death. Like Emily, American lit's most notable self-isolator, I've made friends with solitude, and learned how, as others have said, "The music is in the silence between the notes." How every song, plaintive or playful, is a love song. How each reaches out to someone. How hope is hopeless, and yet, in its mix of happiness and sadness, sublime. How we laugh and cry. How we live and die. How somewhere over the rainbow bluebirds fly.

So I keep on, trying to sing my fears away, I suppose. I've got "Danny Boy" down pat, and I'm working on "In the Garden." It's a hymn I first heard sung at my mother's funeral, when I was ten, so many years ago. It sticks with me. I'm trying to see how to play and sing it with feeling. I'm still on the first verse, which begins with, "I come to the garden alone, while the dew is still on the roses," and ends with, "The joy we share as we tarry there, none other has ever known."

Maybe the first verse is all I'll learn. In these days of death and disease and quarantine and social distancing, I feel it's all I need to know. That we are as one, an indomitable human spirit, with songs, and wings.

Dion Kempthorne was born in Milwaukee and raised in tiny Rewey, Wisconsin. Now a professor emeritus, he lives in the woods in Richland County and imagines he's a young poet.

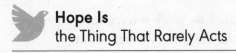

Hope Is
the Thing That Rarely Acts

LISA KRAWCZYK

Hope is the thing that parades
along the street a convincing
show of solidarity rarely
reckoning with what the song

demands. The firefighter leans
outside the fire truck's window,
flicking a cigarette; the last
memory you have on the bus.

The Irish-American's stomping
the St. Patty's parade; oblivious
to the pandemic starting, their bagpipes
screaming into the afternoon

down 29th Street. Lulling Hope to a slow
pace, we now sing falsely Hope's
praises. Until we answer
to her song, we will never

understand Hope's true call.

Lisa Krawczyk (they/them) is a queer, nonbinary poet based in the Midwest. Their poetry can be found in *West Review, In Parentheses, Defunkt
Magazine, One Art Poetry, Vaine Magazine,* and elsewhere. They teach
virtual classes for Gris Literatura.

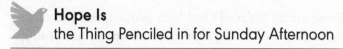

Hope Is
the Thing Penciled in for Sunday Afternoon

COURTNEY KUEPPERS

Sundays have a reputation for being scary, but for me, they are sacred. Not because I go to church—I usually do not. (Sorry, mom and dad.) But because the seventh day of the week (or is it the first? I can never remember) tends to be completely devoid of obligations.

You remember obligations, don't you? Friends' birthday gatherings; professional happy hours; that play you bought tickets to months ago and now somehow the date has snuck up on you. The kind of plans that feel great to make and even better to break—or at least they used to.

Now, these sound like things to daydream about from our separate bunkers, formerly known as living rooms, as we stare out the window at the afternoon sun, hoping a cardinal pays us a visit today. But in the chaos of the busy lives we once lived, the weight of our many obligations could quickly feel heavy.

In the world BC (before coronavirus), I carefully made sure to not commit to any such events on Sundays. The occasional brunch or hike with a pal was sometimes permissible in the morning hours, but come noon—I might as well have turned into a pumpkin.

It was my little retreat from the world. A time I fiercely guarded as my own. A chance to reset before the week ahead.

Now, the need for this refuge seems less necessary—at least not in one designated chunk of time. Lately, as I shelter in place, YouTube yoga practices have replaced the time I once spent in traffic. Home-cooked meals have taken the place of the premade kale salad I once scarfed down for lunch five days a week. While I take a stroll in the afternoons, I call my friends to check in on how they're feeling.

These are all luxuries I feel both grateful, and sometimes guilty, to be experiencing right now. It's not all hunky-dory: I have lost many hours of sleep to anxiety about what the future will or will not look like. But for the most part, I know I have immense privilege right now, in an undeniably scary and uncertain time. My days may lack clear boundaries between work and personal time, but they also somehow feel more balanced.

However, the shift left me with a hole in my once strict schedule: what to do with Sunday afternoons? The answer is at once both retro and completely of the moment: family time.

These days, we gather on Sunday afternoons with a little help from our new friend Zoom. Bridging the miles between my Atlanta apartment and my Midwestern roots, we come together for game night.

First it was charades, then Kueppers-family *Jeopardy*, which required knowledge of family history and memories of childhood trips in order to be victorious. There's been an in-house scavenger hunt, a couple rounds of "categories" and Boggle. I'm happy to report that our fierce sense of competition, penchant for sarcasm, and deep love for one another translates just fine via video chat.

As we laugh, talk about the state of the world, and sip beers from our respective homes, I wonder why we haven't always made this a priority.

For right now, it's the only standing social commitment I have on my calendar every week: right there on Sunday afternoons.

Courtney Kueppers is a writer and journalist. She's originally from the Twin Cities, attended the University of Wisconsin–Eau Claire, and formerly worked for the Eau Claire *Leader-Telegram* and Wisconsin Public Radio.

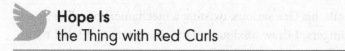

Hope Is
the Thing with Red Curls

CHARLOTTE KUPSH

Hope enters my Zoom conference room sometime after 10:30 at night: red curls and a smile that breaks across a serious face. I've been alone in my apartment for four days, I've had a glass of wine and three (four?) negronis, and rules have ceased to be relevant, so I've invited a man from an app on a digital first date. Hope is the way he sees I'm drunk but takes me seriously anyway, asking about my parents, how I'm doing, whether I want to take a walk tomorrow.

A friend brings me lemon-infused simple syrup, fresh mint from her garden, and a purple, fragrant plant. "I've been buying plants to cope," she says. We never meant to end up here, on this wide-open plain where wind and weather and viruses rip across in what feels like only minutes. The syrup and the mint are to make gin cocktails. The plant is for me.

Hope is driving out to Forty-eighth Street and parking behind Mo Java, a coffee shop that will close by this time next week. Red hair spirals out the front of a knit cap. A Columbia jacket, a soft, calm voice that talks and asks and prompts for three hours while we walk circles around the dilapidated houses north of Nebraska Wesleyan. Hope is the cautious space we hold between our bodies.

Text messages from loved ones beam through the sunny windows of my studio: "Tell me something happy about today." "I'm worried about you." "Call me!" A friend shows up at my door with groceries: eggs, almond milk, sweet potatoes.

Hope is morning coffee in front of my laptop, red curls exploding across the screen. There are Halloween lights strung up in his background. He has a Cafe du Monde mug, and I have Cafe du Monde coffee. I show him my map of Lincoln's recreational trails, the ones I've run on colored in. He answers work e-mails, his face serious, twisting a mechanical pencil between his fingers. I draw anxious, angry characters and label them: "Day 8 of social distancing."

At times, especially at night, hope's knees begin to buckle. "Can you talk? I need someone." "I think I have a fever." My mattress is wearing out from the way I roll across it over and over. "I feel alone." We all cling tightly to its arms; we hoist hope up.

Hope is setting up our camp chairs in the grass outside my apartment building, measured six feet apart by tape measure. We wrap up in fleece blankets and drink beer, the LED camping lamp my dad made me take "for emergencies" illuminating a red beard. It's harder to hear his soft voice from this distance; I make myself quieter, stiller. We talk about breweries, bar hopping, and other things we might do one day, maybe. We listen to the birds and point out the bats, their rapidly flapping wings making jittery, uncertain trails across the sky.

Charlotte Kupsh is a teacher, writer, and doctoral student in composition and rhetoric. Originally from the Driftless region of southwest Wisconsin, she now lives in Lincoln, Nebraska.

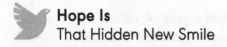

Hope Is
That Hidden New Smile

MATTHEW LARSON

Walking into the lab of our orthodontic clinic, one immediately notices rows of organized 3D-printed models of teeth waiting for fabrication of orthodontic appliances. Most correspond to a patient in braces waiting for retainers so that braces can come off soon. Checking those models is one of my favorite non-clinical activities, because I know the excitement that is coming soon when the new smile is revealed.

Yet when COVID-19 struck—and it became clear that we wouldn't be removing any braces for a while—those models become a lot less exciting.

Owning a small business in dentistry always has a number of stresses: managing treatment, patient interactions, efficient workflow, staffing, marketing, and the list goes on. Never could I have imagined adding required closures, shortage of masks and gloves, inconsistent shipping, and quarantine periods to that list. Constant updates to the recommendations made everything even more challenging.

Creating a plan for our business with the entire landscape constantly shifting created an immensely stressful and busy period . . . where minimal actual orthodontic work occurred.

Although our two-month delay in revealing any new smiles was far from ideal, I still found reason to smile myself. With me out of work and my kids out of school, the world's momentary pause afforded us some much-needed family time. Maybe too much family time, as evidenced by my seven-year-old daughter's new favorite pastime of beating me at cribbage.

Yet professionally, the trials continued. With more time on our hands, we committed ourselves back at the office to help however we could. Although we have always kept high standards for infection control, the guidelines kept changing and required masks were in short supply. We utilized our 3D printer to print masks after dentists across the world came together to design innovative solutions that could be manufactured in-office. I revisited my old woodworking skills to design and build plexiglass dividers to increase safety at the office. We missed our patients and did everything we could to ensure we could safely see each other again.

Finally, although I never expected to be closed for an unknown length of time, I also never expected such a positive response from our patients once we opened. Everyone understood the changes that had to be made for the community's safety. Strangely, the excursion out of the house to the orthodontist became the social highlight of many people's week!

Thankfully, we are now fortunate to see those new smiles daily in our office again. Catching up with all our patients was a different type of stress, but one we approached with a newfound appreciation for how blessed we are to have the privilege to serve them. These days, masks regularly hide those new smiles. But we look forward to the day they won't be hidden any longer and those smiles can again brighten our world.

Matthew Larson is a board-certified orthodontist and co-owner of Larson Orthodontic Specialists in Eau Claire.

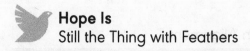

Hope Is
Still the Thing with Feathers

ESTELLA LAUTER

Hope is the ruby-throated
hummingbird who comes
mid-May to look for food
where it had been last fall.

His faded feeder is not
yet there, so he checks
the seed and suet, then flies
into the greening leaves.

Within the hour, my mate
inside prepares the sugared
water in its sterile bottle
to tide him over to the flowers.

We wait, not patiently,
but sure enough, a day
later he comes again
flying straight to the right

spot and perching there
for a long comforting drink
of nectar. Then, the very
next day, there are two.

After retiring from the University of Wisconsin–Oshkosh, **Estella Lauter** has reveled in Wisconsin's writing community. She has published four chapbooks, received several awards, and served as Door County poet laureate from 2013 to 2015.

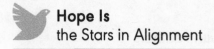

Hope Is
the Stars in Alignment

KAREN LOEB

1. *Osaka map*—
In Osaka, surrounded by skyscrapers
we are lost in crowds on the sidewalk.
My husband finds an open patch of sky
and gazes upward, locating the sun.
"We want to go this way,"
he assures me, leading us
to the elusive Keihan Railway station.

2. *By chance*—
The stars are in alignment
when we cross Sanjo Dori
that busy intersection in Kyoto.
Only back in Japan twenty-four hours
and there's our friend Yuko
among a throng at lunchtime.
We spy her in the hubbub—
white fluffy jacket, face bubbly
with smiles as she spots us.

3. *It's always cloudy*—
I'm told. Fuji-san, as the mountain
is called—perpetually shrouded in clouds.
Never expect a good photo, I've heard.
As the bullet train brings us in sight

Mt. Fuji rises through the mist
as clear and bright as a Hiroshige image.
I snap the picture with my tiny Canon,
and I carry it in my heart today.

Karen Loeb's time in Japan twenty years ago has given her hope and
solace during the time of COVID. These are postcard-type poems she
has written reflecting on that earlier time. Her two-year stint as Eau Claire
writer-in-residence finished in May 2020.

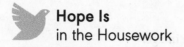

Hope Is
in the Housework

ALLYSON LOOMIS

Late spring morning, 2020, and it's like this: the trees rustle their electric green crinolines; in a patch of sunshine, our cat dreams the snap of songbird bones; the kids sleep late; the dogs frisk around the backyard, paws heavy with mud. Up in the attic, Jon strums an acoustic; down in the kitchen, I wrap my hands around a coffee cup. Worry stirs at the window, on the doorstep, in the dark throat of the heating vent.

Tens of thousands have died in this pandemic. Somewhere, someone is dying right now, without his dear ones there to hold his hand.

What to do? Try this.

The dishwasher wants unloading, and there's fruit to cut up for the kids. The dogs need feeding, and their doggie feet, cleaning. Wipe down those paws; take the dirty towels up to soak in the tub; switch last night's wash to the drier, first picking the lint from the screen. Pile in a new load, then collect the trash from bedrooms and bathrooms, consolidate it down in the kitchen can, and since there's enough room left in the bag, go change the cat box, then tie the Hefty and drag the whole business out to the big green stinker beside the garage, tromp back across the soggy grass to the kitchen, wash the hands, nuke the coffee, crack a quartet of eggs into a bowl, and wipe the counter.

This is not merely a strategy for self-distraction. (Note: it is, in fact, hard not to think of Trump and his shit-weasel minions while dumping the cat box.) No. This is housework. This is real life—my life and your life.

Poke each egg in its eye with a fork, add a pinch of salt, a grind of pepper, and whip that mixture with a burst of energy otherwise only known to rabbits. Flick a knob of soft butter into the iron skillet and light the old stove with a match. These

110

kitchen moves are habitual, precise. Everything you and I do at the stove, at the sink, at the cutting board, we have done a zillion times, because—my god—there's a lot of kitchen work in life, an endless cycle of planning and shopping, chopping and stirring, serving and washing.

I teach full-time at the local university, yet I still feel as though I spend most of my days cooking and cleaning, making this house a home, nourishing its inhabitants. Everyone in my family pitches in—always sometimes, kinda sorta, mostly maybe. Still, there remains a great deal of daily picking-up and putting-away, n'est ce pas? Socks, shoes, jackets, dog toys, game pieces, snack wrappers, tissues, school papers, hair clips, pencils, keys, books, receipts, and sunglasses—this stuff doesn't litter the house all by itself.

I could complain. I have complained. My education was expensive. My talents are few but existent. I've never supposed that anyone, facing death, would wish she could have done more housework.

But during the murky, stretchy days of this quarantine, while all the news is bad, while peril shadows the very passage of time, I find that housework is all I want to do. Cook the meal, serve the meal, scrape the plates. *This is life.* Wash the clothes, dry the clothes, fold the clothes. *Keep it moving.* This housework, this cyclical caretaking in the face of uncertainly must go on as it has always gone on—one era to the next, one season to the next, one day to the next. Don't diminish its importance, my friends: housework is nothing less than a death-defying, continuous, and continuing spiral of love.

So, set out the placemats and pour the milk. The children have awakened, and they are coming downstairs.

Allyson Loomis teaches creative writing at the University of Wisconsin-Eau Claire and writes and publishes fiction and nonfiction, now and again. Currently she is at work on a novel.

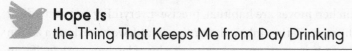

Hope Is
the Thing That Keeps Me from Day Drinking

JON LOOMIS

During the almost three months, now, that we've been social distancing, I've been allowing myself a good-sized martini pretty much every evening around six o'clock. I'm a high-end vodka man who believes a martini should be dry as dust, shaken, not stirred—the full James Bond—and garnished with two pimento olives like green, amphibian eyeballs staring up from the chilly depths. None of these new-fangled garlic or jalapeño or, God forbid, cheese-stuffed olives, thank you very much. Just as there's no crying in baseball, there's no damn cheese in a martini—not ever. So, you get the picture—most evenings, a largeish martini, generally followed by a glass of wine with dinner. At which point, I stop—because Allyson, my wife, tells me to, and I know her to be a person of superior judgment when it comes to things I should or shouldn't do. "You're going to need that liver when you're seventy," she says, or words to that effect. The implication being, of course, that one hopes to stick around that long (I'm sixty-one at this writing, and as far as I know my liver still has a few miles left on it), and that presumably there will be something to stick around for. Hope, in other words, for a brighter future.

Because, let's face it, things are pretty bad right now. Maybe not Great-Depression-and-World-War-II bad, or even (quite) RFK-and-MLK-assassinations-widespread-and-bloody-rioting-'68–'69-flu-pandemic-Vietnam-and-Nixon bad—but still inarguably terrible. I mean, there's just no way to pretend anymore that the chaos, incompetence, and corruption of the Trump administration, plus the pandemic in which, as of today, more than one hundred and thirteen thousand Americans have died, plus mass unemployment and economic paralysis, plus nationwide protests triggered by deep-rooted, systemic police brutality against Black people, plus the (are you kidding me with this?) murder hornets, plus plus plus, aren't just one giant fucking hairball of terrible. We may not have reached Biblical proportions yet, but it feels like we're pretty close.

So, yes—I'm self-medicating. A little. Within certain parameters. There are two reasons for this, beyond the obvious, pleasant mental fuzziness a good martini can induce. First—when my paternal grandmother turned eighty-five, she was in excellent physical health for someone her age. Still, her doctor advised her to take a tall scotch and soda every day at five o'clock, without fail. "People your age need something to look forward to," he said. He understood about biorhythms before the word had been invented—the tendency we humans have to subside into a physical and emotional trough as the sun goes down, particularly in old age. So, instead—a little celebration! And as it turned out, my grandmother lived to an astonishing 106, defying the otherwise terrible genetics of my father's side of the family. That doctor knew his stuff. And while I'm not eighty-five, I, too, need something to look forward to at the end of another pandemic day. The second thing is the ritual. The shaker. The ice. The careful measure (okay, I'm lying here—I don't actually measure). The inspiring rattle and slosh, the few swirled drops of vermouth coating the stemmed glass—the exuberant pour, the plop of the cheese-less, garlic-less, jalapeño-less olives, et voilà! Or, as we say here in Wisconsin—walla! There's much to be said for the orderly business of it all—the careful steps, faithfully followed, that remind us we're not living in a cave (yet), that civilization, or what passes for it now, still lurches along. You'll know it's the apocalypse when I switch to Jäger shots.

But then, as I say, I stop. More or less. And I don't start until the appointed hour, usually. Because yes, I'm planning to continue on with liver number one for a space. Because I can still imagine a better future—a Trump-less, COVID-less future. A less hateful and reactionary future. A more just and, dare I say it, loving future. As the current protest movement unfolds, I'm hopeful that reason and compassion may still have a place in this country. I can imagine the possibility, anyway, if not the promise, as we stagger ahead—two steps forward and one step back, as we always have. If I couldn't—if the only imaginable future was this, where we are right now, the US in June of 2020—there wouldn't be much to celebrate, and there also wouldn't be much point in moderation, either. Over the teeth and past the gums, as my father used to say—watch out, liver, here it comes!

Jon Loomis is a professor of creative writing at the University of Wisconsin-Eau Claire. He is the author of three books of poems and three crime novels. He lives with his family in Eau Claire.

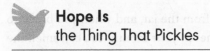

Hope Is
the Thing That Pickles

YIA LOR

Hope is the thing that soaks patiently in vinegar brine. You forget it's waiting in the basement next to the cobwebs and crickets. Spiders, you get, but crickets? You still don't know how they find their way inside. At least their music chirps you to sleep on summer nights, though you must sweep what's left in the fall.

It's not until your favorite restaurant sits empty, your sister is laid off, and yellow tape drapes along the playground equipment that you decide maybe it's time to finally paint the spare room. *Steamed milk*, like the master bedroom. Are paint stores still open? You're not sure but also don't check.

Then you remember the leftover paint from when you did the master bedroom a few years ago. You don't know the rules to painting. Does it expire? You will not have enough for even one wall, but you are desperate for something to keep you from holding your breath, so you will use the old paint regardless of the rules.

In the basement, you find yourself next to the water heater, webs, and crickets. So many. The shelves are mostly empty, except for the can of paint with its lid clearly not shut. That can't be good. You are desperate, though, so you grab the can anyway.

Then you see the jar hidden behind a box full of lids and rings. It's dated July 21, 2019. You pickled on your anniversary, and you know right away it wasn't Nick's idea. You decide to hold off on painting and bring the jar upstairs. You wipe off the dust and webs. Thank goodness, there are no crickets. You take a butter knife along the edge of the lid and pop it open. Bits of dill, onion, garlic cloves, red pepper flakes, and whole black peppercorns sit on top of pinkie-sized pieces of hope that Mama helped you pick after you complained of the sticky summer heat and how it would surely kill you. It did not.

You grab a bit of hope from the jar, and when you bite into it, there is a burst of summer in your mouth. You can smell the tangled cucumber vines and your brother grilling another feast. The kids are taking turns on the tree swings Papa set up a few years ago. Your sisters are mixing bean thread noodles with cabbage, and you're wondering why it's always the hottest day when your family gathers to fry a couple hundred egg rolls.

This summer, hope will grow despite what happens. You and Mama will spend early mornings picking little prickly pieces of it before the sun rises too high. You'll stuff it into many, many jars, and you'll wonder why you always grow so much hope. You'll give most away before the holidays, and sometime when the end of winter rolls around or even into spring, you'll have forgotten that last jar sitting in the dark basement with the cobwebs and crickets.

Yia Lor is a writer and storyteller from Eau Claire. She has served on the advisory board for the Chippewa Valley Writers Guild. She enjoys spending her spare time with family, her yoga mat, and many houseplants.

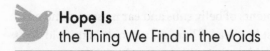

Hope Is
the Thing We Find in the Voids

DAN LYKSETT

Last night, walking the old dog, her gray muzzle pressed against the moldering leaves and grass just now emerging from their snowpack burial. At this moment all life in that ground is microscopic, invisible to me. But it is there. And if I wait through a few more turns of my world on its axis, the sun's warmth will call the visible greening to life. I need only wait a few more turns of my world on its axis.

Deep, black night, no moon but living stars you know from astronomy may be just coming to life or dying or already dead but nonetheless offer their brilliance. No planes overhead, no blinking lights and no distant hum of jet engines, no travelers heading for Chicago with sales orders to be filled or back to Minneapolis with their straw sombreros, happily exhausted from their warm climes' vacations. I recall another night standing on this very ground with the dark sky bereft of planes, September 11, 2001. But the moving night lights and distant hum of jet engines eventually returned to that empty sky. I'm sure they will again. I need only wait for a few more turns of my world on its axis.

The old dog gives me the eye and points her gray muzzle back toward the house. She knows it is time for a treat. Just like she knows when it's time for breakfast, and time for a nap, and time for a walk, and then another nap, and then dinner and another walk and then a treat and then to curl up at the foot of our bed and dream of chasing or being chased.

Throw in moments of belly rubs and ear massages and a lap where she can rest her head. There are no voids in this old dog's life. It is how this old dog's world turns on its axis. I need to be patient. I need only wait for a few more turns of my world on its axis.

Dan Lyksett is a retired journalist who lives south of Eau Claire with his wife, Lisa Van Vleet, a pack of Labrador retrievers, a pug named Ray, and a cat named Norm. After journalism, to keep his tools sharp, he turned to writing fiction and essays.

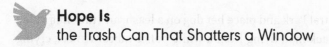

Hope Is
the Trash Can That Shatters a Window

DONTE McFADDEN

Spike Lee's *Do The Right Thing*, released in theaters thirty-one summers ago, sparked what would become my lifelong interest in film. In the film's climactic moment, Mookie throws a trash can through the picture window of the pizzeria where he works. Initially portrayed as a middleman who wants to get paid, he performs this action with a purpose that had not been seen from him up until this point. His friend, Radio Raheem, blasts Public Enemy's "Fight the Power" throughout the narrative as his personal anthem of survival and stature. Earlier in the film, he plays the song at maximum volume in Sal's pizzeria, while Sal furiously demands that he turn it off if he wants to be served. Later, before Sal closes, Radio Raheem returns with two other characters, Buggin' Out and Smiley, in their attempts to shut the pizzeria down over a display of famous "American Italians" on the pizzeria's wall. After a heated exchange littered with racial and ethnic slurs, Sal takes his bat and smashes Radio Raheem's treasured boombox. Radio Raheem then grabs Sal and proceeds to choke him until NYPD officers arrive. The officers take Radio Raheem and place him in a chokehold to the point of his death, leading to Mookie's uncharacteristic outburst.

Do The Right Thing uses blistering heat as a metaphor for racial, ethnic, and class tensions in Brooklyn and throughout New York City. It is easy to force a convenient metaphor between the oppressive heat that absorbs people against their will and the invisible enemy called COVID-19 that confronts us now. It has been nearly a month since the country reached the malevolent milestone of one hundred thousand people who died from this epidemic. This was succeeded by a deadly one-two punch of anti-Blackness: the threat of a white woman calling in a false report on a Black man in response to his request to adhere to the rules

119

of Central Park and place her dog on a leash; and the snuff video of a Black man dying from a white police officer's kneel, crying for his mother as if he knew he was not far from his final breath. Mookie's defiant act of throwing a trash can through the window of his place of employment was not absent of a catalyst, which can also be said about the millions of people throughout the United States and various parts of the world who took part in protests in honor of the lives lost to violent police misconduct and the systemic racism that excuses it. These catalysts came in the form of those two videos that became ingrained in the nation's subconsciousness through a nightmarish loop. Roughly two weeks prior, many of these people saw a video of Ahmaud Arbery turn from a neighborhood jogger to hunted prey, which coincided with the emerging news that Louisville Metro Police Department shot and killed EMT Breonna Taylor while executing a no-knock warrant in pursuit of someone who did not live at that address and who was later learned to already be in custody.

Mookie gains a sense of purpose at the end of the film, yet it took witnessing his best friend dying to gain some clarity. Similarly, these real-life videos were enraging catalysts that prompted people in this country and throughout the world to take their proverbial trash cans and shatter the phone screens that repeated these haunting demises.

The tragic irony about the yellow brick road that leads to hope is that there are bodies buried beneath the pavement—bodies of people who died at the hands of systemic injustices and of a global pandemic. The hope is that when we reach the final destination, vanity is discarded. The hope in this time of COVID-19 is that these lives are not lost in vain.

Born and raised in Milwaukee, **Donte McFadden** is the senior associate director for Undergraduate Research and High Impact Practices for the Educational Opportunity Program at Marquette University. Since 2014, he has been a programmer for the Black Lens Program as part of the Milwaukee Film Festival.

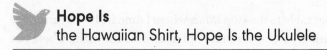

Hope Is
the Hawaiian Shirt, Hope Is the Ukulele

REBECCA MEACHAM

From the edge of our backyard woods, turkeys stroll the greening grass, dripping April rain.

Once, when my husband and I brought our second daughter home, we couldn't picture another baby in the house. *Two kids under two?* we fretted. *How do people do it?* Then we pulled into our driveway where a turkey couple strolled with nineteen fuzzy fledglings.

Nineteen! we counted. And we kept counting as spring turned into summer, then fall. We counted nineteen that stayed together as cars sped by and owls hooted from predatory perches, nineteen as my husband and I fumbled the double stroller, chasing after a toddler while soothing the world's hungriest newborn.

Then, hope was literally a thing with feathers—nineteen things, in fact. Outside, hope took ungainly wing and gobble-gobbled from the trees. Inside, hope stomped floors in our toddler's light-up sneakers, hope strapped itself to my husband's chest in a Baby Björn and kicked its fat baby legs, hope leashed my wrist to a running stroller. Hope threaded through our matching campaign shirts as we watched Barack Obama's first inauguration.

Oh, the audacity of that hope.

They've grown—those birds, our birds—and now the world we've made for them seethes with viral fevers. On Facebook Live, old white men warn of droplets and old white men deny droplets and old white men wear masks and old white men mock masks. Our daughters nest all day in bed, clicking through moved-online schoolwork and snapchatting their squads, their own loud flocks now out of sync and scattered over zip codes. Their teachers try their best. I get it. I've moved my workshops from seminar table to desktop iMac, where I tune in, live, wearing the increasingly weird T-shirts I order late into the night, where our once rambling, funny class discussions are bingo-carded into "raise hand," "join," and "mute." My husband, a college dean, powers through problems of kilns and chorales as students violate apartment noise rules to practice oboe and students sit in hometown parking lots to take exams on iPhones. My mother, at eighty, loathes the thought of her fragility, so we add vocabulary to the language of our eternal compromise: senior hours, curbside pickup, double-layer masking, sanitize, aerosolize, spread.

And yet, our house is a gilded cage that I secretly adore. We're all here, together, my family, in love, in health, alive. It's unspeakable—it's a kind of gluttony, I know—to feel contentment amidst so much grief and misery.

But listen: from her bedroom, our teenager plucks her ukulele and sings about boys she may or may not decide, someday, to love. Her voice is strong and bright and constant.

And look: where there once wailed a newborn, a tween waits for our daily coffee run. She's put on lipstick. She wears a new Hawaiian shirt. She will never step foot from the car.

Outside, the turkeys huddle together and shake off the rain. Inside, our hope sheds and grows like plumage.

Rebecca Meacham is the author of two award-winning fiction collections. A professor of English at the University of Wisconsin–Green Bay, she is the founder of the UWGB Teaching Press and directs the Writing and Applied Arts BFA program.

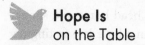

Hope Is
on the Table

CURT MEINE

My first stop this morning is the Tower Rock Farmstead Bakery, where Alma and her crew grow and mill a variety of grains and sell flour, bread, and other baked goods. Their kitchen and shop are squeezed between the house and barn on the farm that has been in the family since the 1870s. They ask their customers to wear masks and to enter one at a time.

My second stop is Straka Meats, a third-generation butcher shop and processor that features locally raised meat. Foot traffic is light at the moment. I enter cautiously, keep my distance, and purchase a box of a dozen chicken breasts.

My third stop is the Cedar Grove Cheese factory. They are especially known for their organic cheese curds, their use of growth-hormone-free milk, and their devotion to ecologically responsible farming. I especially like their baby swiss and mozzarella. They have closed their retail space but offer curbside pickup.

My fourth stop is Enos Farms. When the coronavirus closed everything down, my friends Erin and Jeremy saw their catering business evaporate overnight. They quickly converted themselves into an online store, selling their own prepared foods and offering other items from their supplier farms. I spot my order in a bag on a table under a tent. We catch up at a social distance.

My last stop is the Cates Family Farm. Just a couple years ago Eric and Kiley took over the farm from Eric's parents, Dick and Kim. Their grass-fed Angus and Jersey cattle are grazed with such care that their stretch of Lowery Creek has recently been upgraded to a Class 1 trout stream. Eric has directed me to pick up my order from a walk-in cooler in the barn. No need to interact directly. But Eric comes walking down the gravel driveway to say hello and give me an update on the imminent birth of their second child.

I could keep going, but it's time to head home and shelter on. And I have work to do; I have been a little late getting my own garden going this spring. It is a comfort to know that, even if my modest production falters, I have these neighbors. All my stops today are within twenty miles of my home. I still go to the grocery store in town, which has done an admirable job of making it as safe as possible to shop there. But I have also made a conscious choice, since the pandemic shadow overcame us, to support local farmers and food processors in my corner of rural south central Wisconsin, even more than before. I give them my dollars and receive their products. But just as important, we exchange encouragement amid vast uncertainty.

The pandemic has brought into precise focus the vulnerabilities in our globalized, industrial food system. Everyone, all across the rural-to-urban continuum, has had to think anew about the sources and supply chains and stores that provide our daily bread—and vegetables and milk, meat and potatoes. And the cries for justice, emanating from tragedy in the neighborhoods of Minneapolis, extending to the far ends of the earth, remind us that food justice and food sovereignty are essential parts, too, of the changes we must make. Our interconnected crises call us to come together, to bring health and wholeness to all our landscapes and waterways and communities—to *ourselves*.

My grocery run, though limited and local, strengthens connections between people and land that have been fading and fraying for decades. It nurtures, however inconspicuously, profound seeds of social change. Even under the darkest conditions, hope grows in all our gardens and pastures, vegetable plots and farmers markets, shops and kitchens. This hope is delicious.

Curt Meine is a conservation biologist, environmental historian, and writer based in Sauk County. He serves as senior fellow with the Aldo Leopold Foundation and the Center for Humans and Nature; as research associate with the International Crane Foundation; and as adjunct associate professor at the University of Wisconsin–Madison.

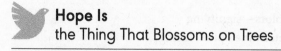

Hope Is
the Thing That Blossoms on Trees

REBECCA MENNECKE

If gravity is a force of attraction,
why does it keep us all so far away
from each other? When Isaac Newton
formed theories of motion, he was alone
at home, avoiding the Bubonic Plague,
the Great Plague, the Black Death
Plague, the *Bring Out Your Dead* Plague

because that's all anyone was back then
before vaccines and hand soap and Purell
that's out of stock anyway. It would be two
hundred years before scientists
determined what bacteria plotted
such a diabolical illness: skin turning black
with blood, filling pores, pouring

onto rat fleas to infect
the next victim. But no one knew
that, back then. Talk about living
in uncertain times. Back then,
there was no twenty-second rule, no six-
foot rule, no limit one toilet paper pack
per customer rule, only the rules

of physics we call *laws*
because they created order
from disorder, which the world probably
needed. And Newton made lots of laws:
creating early calculus while his room
was lit by candles instead of electricity,
looking through prisms to study

refractions of colors—signifying
promise—to determine optics, lazing
beneath a tree and thinking how
all motion leads downward
or repels. Infinitesimal calculus
is the study of continuous
change, so what Newton really

hypothesized is a theory of
life because everything is changing:
plane fumes aren't soaring so high
above ground like they used to,
the rivers in Italy look like water,
real water, & less gas in the sky
from cars mean people can breathe,

and everyone applauds the guy
who works at Walmart because finally,
finally, we all see how his work is good
too, & I have to wonder, sitting at home
like Isaac Newton, quarantined and self-
isolated in self-pity while new
plagues ravage cities where I grew

up, eating everyone in the world whole:
if every action has an equal and opposite
reaction, then the budding growths
on the trees outside my window—
as the sky pours down
my windowsill—well, they must
be the Earth's form of
        balance.

Rebecca Mennecke is the associate editor of *Volume One*, a poetry
reader at *The Adroit Journal*, and a writer. She lives in Eau Claire with her
black cat, Cuttlefish.

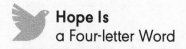
Hope Is
a Four-letter Word

OSCAR MIRELES

Hope is a four-letter word.

All the other four-letter words
have a certain way
of breeding familiarity with shock.

Webster's dictionary defines a four-letter word as
"any of several short words
regarded as coarse or offensive."

Hope gives you nine points in Scrabble.
Four points for the *h*
one point for the *o* and *e*
and three points for the *p*.

I was surprised to find *jazz* and *jizz* are both four-letter words
and get you twenty-nine points each in Scrabble
as I was doing research for this poem.

The letter *h* in hope is symbolic of the home life.

H is also symbolic of the flow of happiness in the energy of it.

I believe hope
can change the direction
of our understanding
of four-letter words

I hope the word hope
becomes the beacon of light
that blinds the darkness
that surrounds us

Hope is a four-letter word

Never forget that

Pledge to never use the other
Four-letter words in public again
Now that's a big hope . . .

Maybe hope has the strength
to bend the universe
to help others
see the world in a new way.

Hope is a four-letter word.

Oscar Mireles is a published poet, the editor of three anthologies, and author of a children's book. He served as Madison poet laureate for two terms, from 2016 to 2020.

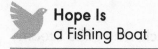

Hope Is
a Fishing Boat

RALPH MURRE

"And our sails are a hopeful color/Filled with the wind of changing times." —*Sylvia Fricker Tyson*

That's right, an old gill-netter out of Gill's Rock, named *Hope*. Should be the name of every fishing boat, maybe. How else do you go out in bad Great Lakes weather except hoping that nets are still there, untorn, hoping you're fishing for more than your fuel, that cormorants left some for you. Hoping there's some left for your son and his son, too. Hoping to stay afloat. And yet you fish.

Hope is every tractor on every farm. The seed. The bank. The soil. The rain. *Was* the corn-picker that took Uncle Ned's arm. Whatever it is or was about sunlight on new-turned earth that first took your heart. Hope is feeling that again. Your son, Ben. Your daughter, Adrienne. For them, you say, you farm.

Hope, dammit, really *is* the thing with feathers. This white-crowned sparrow outside my window this dismal day, whatever crumbs may come its way, whatever love another sparrow gives. Hope is the only thing I see that feeds the gnarled cedar on the limestone cliff where it lives. Hope is the six-year-old you, your first ride on a two-wheeler. The seventy-six-year-old you and every ride on a BSA, or a Duo-Glide.

Hope is what's left when panic and pandemic take a world from which hope has been torn.

Just now, out there, a pair of orioles, dressed in what may be the most hopeful color.

Just now, in here, an assurance that hope still *is*, even in the wind of changing times.

Ralph Murre has spent much of the last three-quarters of a century along Wisconsin's east coast. A jack-of-all-trades and writer, he served as Door County poet laureate from 2015 to 2017.

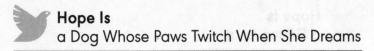

Hope Is
a Dog Whose Paws Twitch When She Dreams

DEBRA PETERSON

The good girl walks easy,
sure-footed on a path she knows by heart.

Her nose, a tuning fork, vibrates
at cracker crumbs on a sidewalk,
stains on a fluttering wrapper,
a soggy tidbit half-buried in slush.

Some days when she pulls hard,
the leash follows her lead.
Some days, a squirrel dashes up a tree;
in her heart, she chases it into the sky.

Under the name Delaney Green, **Debra Peterson** writes long and short
works of speculative fiction. She has worked as a reporter, copy editor,
professional actress, teacher, farm laborer, and, lately, mask-sewer.

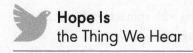

Hope Is
the Thing We Hear

JESSI PETERSON

Hope is the thing
we hear, or in this case don't
when the traffic noise from Highway 29
no longer follows the curvature of the hills,
singing down slopes, channeling
down ravines to reach us.

Hope is what we are listening for now,
the rippling trill of the crane's return,
often flying too far up to be seen.

The soft sough of wind through the feathers
of swans as they aim for pooled snowmelt
in the fields west of town, a spot
to rest, to glean like Ruth
what's left of last year's harvest.

The late night yodel and yip of coyotes
from the prairie floodplain along the river,
already such consummate artists
at social distancing they hear me crack
our patio door a quarter mile away
and clam up.

The rumble of a neighbor's truck, dropping off
a widow's portion of wood for my mother's woodstove
but not dropping in.

The almost silent rasp of my pet snail eating,
just out of estivation while we go in,

his retractable teeth contending with spinach and waiting
for the grass I planted in his cage today to sprout.

Waiting like the rest of us, taking things at the pace he knows
that we don't know yet.

Jessi Peterson lives on her family's farm on the Chippewa River near
Eau Claire and works as a children's librarian. She is a poetry reader
for the literary journal *Barstow & Grand* and lives in a hand-built cord-
wood hobbit house with one husband, two cats, and many, many, many
books.

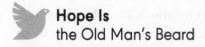

Hope Is
the Old Man's Beard

TY PHELPS

One afternoon, I wrote about gray. Gray will take you places. Gray is the faded snow of a Wisconsin February piled high in a shopping mall parking lot, speckled with exhaust. It's certain eyes in a certain light, or, occasionally, the Big Lake, or wolves, though their shading is more of a confluence of black and white and in-betweenness. Like the granite that heaves itself out along the North Shore, Precambrian bedrock birthed 2.7 billion years ago. Or lichen that clings to the rock, or Usnea, another sort, the Old Man's Beard, climbing grayish-green in the trees.

You can follow your gray thoughts and arrive in these ghost woods, each tree a universe of messy living, each wisp of the Old Man's Beard a fractal thread to somewhere else.

Lichen is the world's weirdest construct. This is science. Part algae, part fungus, two biological kingdoms combining into a single living organism. They're debating if bacteria is in the mix too, which would bring the kingdom total to three. Lichen is like if humans were also trees but were still humans but were really trees, cellulose and -lite blending into some newness, lungs and limbs and photosynthesis on a razor's edge of liminal life, a stuck-between, a spread-across.

Old Man's Beard is the color of a long, lonely Sunday afternoon where time stretches out in front of you and you're too sad to nap, too despondent to talk, too brain-tired to read or write or create. It's the color of all the time, right now. Or it's possibly not.

Have you seen it? It's beautiful. The way it clings, wispy, to tree trunks. It grows in tassels, up to twenty centimeters long. Some think it kills trees, but it's only seizing opportunity when trees go leafless, stepping into the void. This is merely how things work. The world is often less beautiful than we want it to be, though sometimes it is better, too.

133

The Old Man's Beard isn't nefarious, though it resembles will-o'-the-wisps hovering in the forests. But it doesn't try to lure you away from your mother, or your lover, or your soul. It is content with its duality in a way so many of us are not. Why is it so hard for humans to be more than one thing at once? We need poets to emerge periodically, muddy and wild, to remind us that this is possible.

Lichen reproduces asexually, but this fact does not necessarily have any bearing on its proclivity for pleasure. Does the Old Man's Beard curl its tendrils around itself? Does it care about friction, in either the physical or metaphorical sense? Does it whisper love notes through the rumor mill of forest-floor mycelium?

I want the Old Man's Beard to become the new decorative gourd. Hung like garlands in homes during holidays. Subject to viral McSweeney's articles. Clumped inside cornucopias. Spilling out as a bounty of hope.

Ty Phelps is a writer, teacher, and musician from Madison. He is an MFA candidate in fiction and nonfiction at Virginia Commonwealth University, where he won the 2019 poetry prize through the Academy of American Poets.

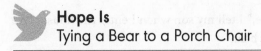
ERIC RASMUSSEN

In the early days of a shelter order, we desire to help, support, entertain, and distract. For a minute I toy with the idea of learning "The Hustle" on harmonica to accompany my son who is learning "The Hustle" on trombone so we can make some hilarious and unbelievably shareable video. My son is not interested in that level of commitment. Honestly, neither am I.

But soon an idea comes across my feed for a community-wide effort that is more our speed. A teddy bear scavenger hunt! Place a bear somewhere visible so families out on walks have something to search for. That is exactly the level of energy expenditure we can handle. My daughter fetches a bear, and the kids and I collaborate over its placement in one of the chairs on the front porch.

A short while later I take my own afternoon walk, and it amazes me how well the teddy bear scavenger hunt accomplishes its goal. Every stuffed animal peeking behind venetian blinds or hanging from a curtain rod is a little inside joke that feels like community. But this is not what gives me hope. I come from a city in a part of the world that usually does a pretty nice job of supporting our neighbors. Not everyone, and not easily, and not always right away, but for the most part, we've got each other's backs.

After my loop around the neighborhood I pass in front of my own house, with my daughter's stuffed animal out front. As far as scavenger hunts go, ours is a bit of a challenge—the bear is the same color as the chair upholstery, and it can only be seen from a certain angle. But another thought occurs to me. Call it the jack-o'-lantern concern. What if a bunch of neighborhood youths decides our bear is ripe for shenanigans?

"Get some rope," I tell my son when I enter the house. "We have to tie up that bear."

This is what gives me hope. Pranksters targeting our teddy bear. People on the internet griping about having to stay inside and arguing about what counts as an essential business. All the testimonials of rampant screen time and day drinking. Without discounting the need to take a pandemic seriously and act with each other in mind, I love that the fear doesn't entirely consume us. The empty roads fill me with confidence that we shall weather this crisis. The occasional car does too.

From the sidewalk, you can't tell that our bear is trussed up like a prisoner in a spy movie, but it's there, representing both our nobler intentions and our basal instincts. We need both to get us through, adorable plush smiles on our faces, and double knots around our necks and paws.

Eric Rasmussen serves as editor of the regional literary journal *Barstow & Grand* and fiction editor of the online journal *Sundog Lit*. He resides in Eau Claire, where he teaches English at Memorial High School.

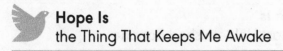

Hope Is
the Thing That Keeps Me Awake

RITA MAE REESE

Hope is the thing
that keeps me awake at night,
a thing that got inside—
I must have left a window
open—and now is making
itself known, asking is this home
with the same small voice
as my daughter asking
when she can play inside
with friends again. Hope is
the gap between her question
and my answer. Hope is the branch
holding the two crows calling and calling
to the smaller crow on the ground,
unable to fly. Hope is the little plate
of seed and apple left nearby. Hope
is saying yes, this is home.

Rita Mae Reese is the author of *The Book of Hulga*. She designs Lesbian Poet Trading Cards for Headmistress Press and is the literary arts director at Arts + Literature Laboratory in Madison.

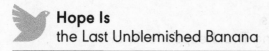

Hope Is
the Last Unblemished Banana

JENNA RINDO

Hope is the last unblemished banana
ripening in a maple hand-turned bowl
found art on the counter hidden from

the oldest daughter thrown into a twitchy
growth spurt—sweet as vanilla wafers

crushed for pie crust one hour
plunged into soft ripe lies the next.

Emily knew *forbidden fruit a flavor has.*
Maybe every fruit has its secret

under thick skin sealed tight against
viral enemies in airborne droplets.

We wait for our direct deposit endorsed
promise—broken or delayed—our balance

tipping into a darker shade of gray-furloughs
ever evolving epicenters–clusters of cases

heavy like a full hand of bananas.
But this morning I will slice this almost ripe

green-tipped finger—spread it with nut butter
arrange the coins into a happy face

on my youngest son's sky blue melamine plate.
The end cone is for me. I sandwich it

between crackers—hiding my craving
for sweet and salty—swallow back a sour
morning aftertaste—carry my secret deep.

Jenna Rindo worked for years as a pediatric intensive care nurse. She now teaches English to speakers of other languages. She and her husband, Ron, raised five children on five acres in rural Pickett, Wisconsin.

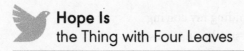
Hope Is
the Thing with Four Leaves

SCOUT ROUX

When lady luck weeps
with her many heads
in the day, taut red stems bent
below the windowpane, I know

to take her to the kitchen sink and watch
until the water comes out the other end
brown, salt soaked, it washes down
the drain.

And soon, how her response gives me
pause: sparse wave
of buds
of green growth rising to the east
folded like hands
in a prayer for peace.

I found my luck someplace local.

When the cashier asked
if I found everything alright
I let her know
with a smile I had
more than I need.

Scout Roux is a Madison-based writer of poetry and fiction whose work has found many loving homes in print across the country. They currently serve as a fiction editor for *Nightingale & Sparrow* magazine.

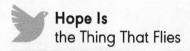

Hope Is
the Thing That Flies

MARGARET ROZGA

Sow as early in spring
as the ground can be worked.
Cool weather crops, lettuce,
spinach. Radishes. Hope
soon sprouts.

Look, distinct green shape
like butterfly wings. Hope—

a butterfly—first
a white dot nearly invisible
on the back of a leaf,
then caterpillar, chrysalis,
wings, the ability to fly,

alight on a flower, pollinate. Hope
now for the fruit
and rain on the radishes.

Dr. Margaret Rozga, professor of English emerita at the University of
Wisconsin-Milwaukee at Waukesha, creates poetry from her ongoing
concern for social justice issues. She was a participant in Milwaukee's
marches for fair housing and later married civil rights leader Father
James Groppi.

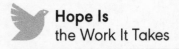

Hope Is
the Work It Takes

RAFAEL FRANCISCO SALAS

Grandma has moved to the farm. My mother's farm, to be clear. You wouldn't assume to encounter a farm managed entirely by the likes of my mom. She is tiny, about four feet ten inches in boots, and will be in her seventieth year this summer. But she is stringy, as strong as anyone I know. To add a nonagenarian matriarch into life on the farm is quirky, like a pairing from a novel.

This all stems from the onslaught of the virus, of course. My family pulled my grandmother out of her retirement facility right before it was locked down. We feel lucky that she is safe, or safer. We hope for the best.

The farm is a refuge. It harbors sheep, dogs, stray cats, stray people. It has been host to barbecues for the NAACP, wedding parties, Thanksgivings, and other gatherings large and small. Mom transformed a life of activism and raising her children into this. It is a sanctuary and she watches over it carefully. She knows the fox that runs in the back field and the migrating birds that stop in from the adjoining marsh. A sanctuary, yes, but one that requires diligence and pragmatism too. You are welcome here unless you are a possum stealing cat food. She has been known to dispatch those with a sledgehammer.

Mom turned a small, failing dairy farm into a streamlined sheep operation. Seventy acres have been converted to no-till grazing for her flock. A federal grant funded permanent fencing and water piped to the length of the property. To her, grazing sheep, a sound fence, and sustainable soil is as close to perfection as one could hope for. She tends fences, helps her ewes bear their lambs, moves snow, fixes equipment. Her fingers are gnarled and arthritic. "Witch's hands," she calls them.

She created this place herself. Her goal was to be a steward of this land, for her animals, for the land itself, and for the people who come here, most recently my grandmother.

When I see Mom and Grandma, now reunited on the farm, I continually think about these strange times. As global and national crises of illness, racial unrest, and political upheaval shake the very foundation of our lives, Mom quietly cares for her own mother, who has reached her twilight. It isn't easy. Grandma may never return to her old life. The farm may be her last home. My mother knows this, and with equanimity offers her hardened hands to tend both her flock and her ailing mother.

Still, they stand together, side by side, tending all they can.

Rafael Francisco Salas is a Wisconsin-based artist. He combines landscape, the legacy of portraiture, architecture, religious iconography, and country music into artwork that evokes a strange, rural poetry. He is a professor of art at Ripon College.

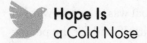

Hope Is
a Cold Nose

KATHERINE SCHNEIDER

When I brought my tenth Seeing Eye dog home from training at the end of January, I knew I had lots of work ahead of me. Calvin (a two-and-a-half-year-old black Lab) and I had trained intensely for nineteen days at The Seeing Eye in New Jersey. We were well bonded and a great team. He trusted me to feed and take care of him, and I trusted him to lead me across busy streets, on and off buses, around obstacles, and to lie quietly in meetings, restaurants, church services, etc. At home we'd begin to hone our skills in navigating in snow and ice and learn my neighborhood and town.

Then COVID-19 hit. Public buildings, churches, and restaurants closed. Meetings happened online instead of in person. People stopped visiting and kept their distance when we passed them on the sidewalk.

I can't do social distancing like sighted people. I can't know if I'm six feet from you, or if I'm standing on the X in the line. When I'm in an unfamiliar situation, I need to hear a verbal greeting like, "Hello, I'm across the street with my dog," instead of receiving a more visual smile or wave. On occasion, I may need to touch things or take an elbow for direction.

Thankfully I encounter these frustrations with my new guide and friend Calvin by my side. When people distance themselves from us, he figures it's their loss. We stick to a schedule, take at least one walk a day, and work on our relationship.

He's 99 percent calm and eager to please but there's 1 percent wildness that comes out at home in a game he's invented. What's the game? He'll grab something he shouldn't have, like a half-full carton of eggs I'd momentarily placed on the floor, and then torment me with it. Picture the carton of eggs sticking out of his jaws as he bumps it against my hand. Then, the game is on! Since some of his grabs have been things that could have made him sick if ingested, I've worked hard on the concept of trading.

You give me the egg carton, and I'll give you this luscious treat.

He's orbiting around the dining table with egg carton in jaws and I'm chasing him with my trade in hand. I have to move calmly, or in his excitement, he'll chomp down on the carton. Eventually a trade is made, and I take the mauled carton into the kitchen. Two eggs are fine, exactly what I needed for the brunch I was preparing, and the rest of the gooey mess goes into the trash. By this point, Calvin is busy licking egg debris off the floor.

"You'd better apologize," I tell him.

He comes and licks my hand, then transmits a look that says, "I'll apologize if you need me to, but put an egg carton on the floor, and I'll do it again!"

My hopes are: Calvin will gradually mature and the crazy chase games will tone down a little—I'm seventy-plus, and soon he'll be three.

I also hope that when the world reopens, Calvin and I will have more opportunities to strengthen our working relationship. As with each of his predecessors, he'll be my best friend, my eyes, and my favorite mode of transportation. His sweetness, intelligence, stubbornness, and teasing make each day a new, joy-filled adventure.

Hope is a cold nose, a good trade, and a team growing stronger every day.

Katherine Schneider is a retired clinical psychologist, blind from birth. She is the author of several books on aging and living with disabilities, most recently *Hope of the Crow: Tales of Occupying Aging*.

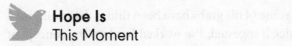

Hope Is
This Moment

TRACY SCHULDT HELIXON

Hope is one cup of sugar
one stick of butter
my pandemic anxiety
firmly packed
brown sugar
applesauce.
Time to mix.
She's eleven now
no longer so excited about this cookie-making business.
At age four, she burst with
delight.
Tonight's motivation is product, not process.
Still, I'll take it,
gratefully.
Two cups of flour
baking soda
salt.
More mixing.
"Good job. Remember to scrape the sides."
She nods.
Hope is when we pour the chips.
She steers the spatula through thick batter,
making sure
chocolatey goodness
reaches
every
single
cookie.
Hope is sliding the tray in the oven,
closing the door,

waiting.
"Smells good!" says my husband.
And her teenage brothers
emerge from their rooms.

Hope
is
this
moment

standing in the kitchen
together,
the five of us
bustling
talking
laughing
pouring milk.
I savor the warmth
and the sweetness
and maybe even
a cookie.

Tracy Schuldt Helixon is a teacher and award-winning author of children's books and historical fiction. She seeks out creativity, goodness, and chocolate and can't stop smiling each time she finds it.

147

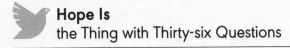

Hope Is
the Thing with Thirty-six Questions

PATTI SEE

I click on "Want to Fall in Love with Your Partner Again? Science Says to Ask Them These 36 Questions" for the same reason I'm wearing pajama pants at noon on a Tuesday: I'm abiding by Safer at Home.

Dr. Arthur Aron's study explored whether intimacy could be developed between two strangers. One group of participants made small talk with a partner; the other group asked each other thirty-six questions that became increasingly more personal. You don't need to be a scientist to figure out who felt more bonded. The results were used to better understand prejudice and to improve relationships between police officers and community members. When shared with a romantic partner, these become part Cosmopolitan quiz, part premarital inventory.

My husband and I sit at our counter with drinks and ask each other some of Aron's questions. Bruce reads aloud, "If you were able to live to the age of ninety and retain either the mind or body of a thirty-year-old for the last sixty years of your life, which would you want?" He smiles: "I know what I'd want . . . for you."

"Like you'd live to see it," I tease back. I read, "Tell your partner what you like about them."

Bruce answers, "You're nice and so competent." I groan. Is this a Yelp review of his favorite dental hygienist?

"Wow," I say sarcastically. "That's something."

"It is," he says. "You're nice to everyone." He adds, "And anyone who knows you knows a little bit about the good things you do, but I know them all."

I tell him, "You always say the right thing to me or to your kids or even to strangers." I tear up.

Crises—like the recent pandemic—create waves of vulnerability that sometimes speed up the usual trajectory of our lives.

148

Consider intense romances during wartime or the children conceived within days of watching the Twin Towers fall. One year from now we could easily count another baby boom or even an uptick in divorces. As social distancing throws us together in ways we didn't expect, what's immeasurable is the evolution of not just romantic bonds but deeper connections among family and friends. Dr. Aron reminds us, "Relationship quality is the biggest predictor of human happiness."

After another drink, Bruce and I take these thirty-six questions to a new level: we choose one and answer how we think the other might. I describe what Bruce would say about his perfect day.

Bruce tells me what he imagines I would want to be famous for. I tell him what I know he'd want: "You're at a small jazz club and someone in the band calls you up onstage from the audience. You sing the crap out of a song."

As the night goes on, Bruce asks, "Shouldn't there be questions on what annoys you about a partner? Or at least something you'd like to change?"

"We'll add our own next time," I say. We have only time and each other on our hands.

Patti See's award-winning work has appeared in numerous national publications and anthologies. She lives in Lake Hallie, Wisconsin, with her husband, writer Bruce Taylor.

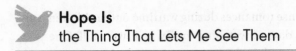

Hope Is
the Thing That Lets Me See Them

KAIA SIMON

"You home?" my sister texts me and then immediately follows with a pair of laughing-crying emojis, because of course I'm home and she knows it. We have nowhere else to be. We aren't really allowed to be anywhere else.

"You betcha!" I reply, tongue in Midwest cheek.

One second later, my Google Hangouts app chimes. I click to join. My brother and my sister appear, each in their own box, be-headphoned and smiling at me from their living rooms. I am so happy to see them.

My sister lives in New Rochelle, New York, the site of one of the first COVID-19 outbreaks in the US. My brother lives in Minneapolis, the last of the three of us to be officially ordered to #StayAtHome. I have never felt so far away from both of them as I do now.

Even though I only want to stare at their faces, I try to remember to stare at the green light next to my webcam when I'm talking to my brother and sister, because that looks like I'm making eye contact with them. And all I want right now is contact.

These daily conversations through our webcams help me focus within the radius of what's most important. We affirm that we are all still symptom-free and feeling good, even if cooped up. While I stare at the webcam light and smile desperately, in my peripheral vision I see my three-year-old niece's quarantine fashion choices of the day. My seven-year-old nephew runs into view and asks me to give him a math problem to solve. "Tía Kaia, I like to add hundreds. So you can give me two numbers that go up to nine hundred and ninety-nine!" He writes the numbers on a folded piece of paper and dashes off camera to solve them. My brother tells us what it's like to be the IT guy while his coworkers try to set up video conferences with clients from their own homes. And all the while I focus on the green webcam light, beaming my love through it, willing it to shine through the laptop screens on the other side, hoping they feel it.

I learned this trick—to make eye contact through the camera instead of by looking at their eyes on the screen—when I was applying for professor jobs a couple of years ago and many search committees did first round interviews over Skype. It felt unnatural then, and it still does now. Now, though, this isn't about projecting a scholarly, put-together self who'd make a great colleague. This is about trying to keep myself steady amid the churn all around me. This is about using a webcam to do with my eyes what my arms cannot: gather my family up close to me, then step back, hold them at arm's length, and squeeze their shoulders to confirm that they, that we, are okay. Until I can do this in person, I will focus on the green light that connects us. I am so grateful to be able to see them these days.

Kaia Simon is a lifelong Wisconsinite (except for her seven-year stint at the University of Illinois in Urbana-Champaign, where she earned her PhD). She is a writer and professor in the English Department at the University of Wisconsin-Eau Claire.

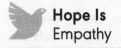

Hope Is
Empathy

DEANNA SINGH

My purpose is to shift power to marginalized communities. One of the most challenging things about my work is getting people who have power to understand why shifting it is essential. To do that work, I lean heavily on storytelling to help people empathize with the underserved.

But there is only one thing that builds empathy better than storytelling, and that is lived experience. In many ways, the COVID-19 pandemic shed light on social inequities. The impact of the virus on our everyday lives has demonstrated what it feels like to be without power amid challenging situations. To illustrate my point, let's look at what happened in the realm of education.

For decades, I have been an ardent advocate for educators, particularly those who work with underserved students. These educators teach students in highly stressful environments, with limited resources, and without the necessary support. They have to also meet the demands of children with varying abilities, behavioral challenges, and the pressure of ever-changing benchmarks. New curriculums show up, and they have to adapt to them quickly. And yet, despite these well-documented challenges, teachers remain underpaid and undervalued. To add insult to injury, when people introduce policies and practices that would help alleviate the challenges our educators face daily, institutions meet them with resistance and little compassion.

But when the schools shuttered because of COVID-19 and our children came home, it became wildly apparent just how much we depend on our educators. When circumstances dropped even a fraction of their responsibilities onto our plates, we saw how difficult their jobs always were. Many parents were at a loss for how to handle their children all day. We did not know how to differentiate learning between children in our home. We did not know how to keep our children focused or how to guide them in their homework. Innumerable Facebook support groups, tweets, and text messages demonstrated just how many people struggled with doing the jobs that our teachers do every day. In short, this lived experience helped shine a light on just how much we rely on our teachers and how important it is that they have the resources to help our children.

Through the shift to distance learning, the challenges of teaching became just one of many things that people are now able to view with more empathy. I hope that as we build what the future looks like, we will not lose the insight that this moment has granted us. The COVID-19 pandemic gave many a glimpse into what it feels like to be under-resourced. Having momentarily experienced relative powerlessness, I hope we will make changes in education and other social institutions to shift power to marginalized communities.

As an expert social entrepreneur, **Deanna Singh** wants to live in a world where marginalized communities have power. She is an accomplished author, educator, business leader, and social justice champion.

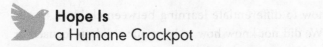

Hope Is
a Humane Crockpot

ABRAHAM SMITH

pick up a stick these days and it's snakes and
here it turns out we'll be just shy
of eternally gone
almost always have been
sewin masks from long gone
grumpy gramsy's quilt stash cock chin
and like the larger birds sing
crazy as 16 '61 dryers fulla frozen blubber
chawin in the attic here in harm nation
it's hard not to thin thinkin
of the body ma as a broken coffeepot
one those old aluminum sneaky light percolator jobs
the rattail hard kids use to scoop rock creek crayfish
trick is they hit the gas in reverse and there ain't
anythin much more human than
our gate great wide shadow circling down
shading cup on up over the sun
bull shake hand what we done can't be undone
people season perpetual storm
phone spine bent platte river sunflower
stuccoed and malicious in snow ices
soon the nose will cut the heart open
and blood will too run circular
hot gold down the throat
reach for the egg under the hen
and that's a snake too
of the bull snake variety can't be blamed
warm is warm is warm is warm even when
yr roof's a dawngonegonzo fidget spinner hey
hey it's jughead egglife ma and i hate to see

you smellin like rubber stood up on
while leg trap snap hearts freak behind
sling wink bar javelin got a boomerang tendency
and in some countries it ain't even new noon
briefest taste watchful jail lights sugar surge weave
we've ez-mail-in made a self
at rat rant expense of all others
dished and steamin you still workin?
tell me when to take it away
it is the eyepatch over yr heart heart
it tar the monsanto tailings oaten in my lowbrow rite shoe
try and dream on that med just try
when alls you see in sleep is seep by some shedding sandstone
and a wolf with a housecat she's
cleanin down to tasty there there
cat come to water it's a selfie life
and we all come to be by so many
i'll be flavor wanders now
who got their mood foot on my loose thread
do the mummy hoodoo nono
radical gratitudes
spurt maggots too
off saddle glad path
was that my sandwich or yr hand?
go book a read backwards
go try flip skinny pages til true wrinkles unski
off the skin and innocences
retread newest dust in america
upheld by trembling peachfuss
robin pronouncin newday
with an umlaut over the dream
of the invention of a first plow
fashioned of hawk's-wing dragged along
the prairie scathed no
unzipt everything no

held shut rooted in as is
only higher sages a little tickled tick the bees off
8 9 seconds when things resettle
it's a picnic of slippery fish
held in place with a kicked can
fulla backwash my earliest memory
i am before grades at the mount there's a patch of grasses
the watcher you kids go collide there
i go to take a drink of pepsi free
and a bumble bee kittens
from the sip hole all bear den sleepy
in a trashsack for clothes
rides her thorn on to who knows
and i begin to arbor uncut the imago
costs you reader pal based off all this
wash of flat rate chat to come
maybe less than the faucet leak whose
rounding pearl gets a gutful and
descends quieter than a sunflower
seed down a ballplayer deep
deep leftfield ol gimpshrimp at the plate
ol dandelion mic the ghostest with the mostest
prays for a kick sing welder bell star
ticktickin swimmin hole
toaded turded teaked teach me
the folded napkin and the sheeting tuck
everything so
hospital perfect
until no it's not

Abraham Smith is the author of six poetry collections and coauthor of a
fiction collection. Originally from Ladysmith, Wisconsin, today he lives in
Ogden, Utah, where he is assistant professor of English and codirector of
creative writing at Weber State University.

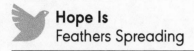
Hope Is
Feathers Spreading

ANGELA SORBY

Let's say it together—
dinosaurs had feathers.

Let's say it until we can picture
the Mink River estuary,

and in it, a heron,
holding its long archaic neck

erect, pinning space
to time and time

to space. Pre-Emily D,
pre-*hominid*, nothing

was alphabetized,
and yet there was a system,

a double helix,
learning and repeating,

learning and repeating,
shrinking therapods,

turning teeth to beaks,
optimizing wings.

Dinosaurs had feathers.
Let's say it together

until we can hear no news,
save the estuarial

water. A heron is news
enough for one summer.

Angela Sorby is professor of English at Marquette University in Milwaukee. She's the author of three poetry books, plus a critical book, an anthology of children's poetry, and an edited collection on poetry and pedagogy.

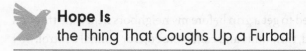

Hope Is
the Thing That Coughs Up a Furball

ERIN STEVENS

On the fifth day of social distancing, I had my first breakdown. Always a rule follower, I was doing a great job of staying away from everyone, mainly because I live alone. It was just me, hanging out on my couch, in my tiny studio apartment, with a fictional series about aliens cued up on Netflix.

Before transporting to Roswell, New Mexico, for the evening, I gave a final scroll through Instagram. It seemed like every post I saw in my feed, every story I tapped on, everyone was with someone else—spouses or partners, family, children, roommates, friends, fugitives being shielded from the law, etc.

Everyone was with someone else but me.

On any other night, my homebody-self would have been like *wow, that's really nice. Good for them!* And then I'd go back to eating Izzy's ice cream and watching an alien fall in love with a human without giving it a second thought.

But this wasn't just another night. This was the first Tuesday night of many that would be spent practicing the art of social distancing, and my mind was busier than normal with its incessant overthinking. Nighttime has a way of tricking us into believing the worst things about ourselves and our situations. The weight of an irrational fear I'd never had before tap-danced like a hippo on my chest. It felt as if heavy words like "quarantine" and "social distancing" and "isolation" were trying to bust down my front door, three thieves in the night trying to steal my peace and my hope.

I am so alone, I thought, over and over and over. For about five long minutes I stared up at my apartment's puckered ceiling and had a very uncute meltdown, letting the feeling of absolute loneliness unravel and weave through me—whether it was true or not didn't matter.

I needed to get a grip before my neighbors heard me through our shared, thin walls and called the cops or animal control. So I got up to make a cup of tea, because what else are you supposed to do when there's an internal and external crisis at hand?

On my way to the kitchen, I almost stepped in a small, fresh pile of cat puke.

Murphy sat next to it, blinking up at me.

"Seriously?" I asked, my voice cracking. "Read the room, man."

More blinking. *How dare you forget about me,* he seemed to say. *I'm here, too.*

I grabbed the roll of paper towel and disinfectant that's always within arm's reach these days, then turned around to clean up the mess.

It was gone.

I looked at Murphy, confused, then repulsed.

"Did you just eat . . ." I started to ask. He answered by cleaning his mouth with his paws. I disinfected the area where I thought the puke had been but couldn't be certain.

"You're so gross," I said to him.

And then I laughed.

Erin Stevens is the proud product of the Kaukauna public school system and graduated from the University of Wisconsin-Eau Claire with degrees in English-Creative Writing and Organizational Communication. She lives in Minneapolis with her cat, Murphy.

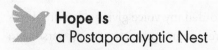
HEATHER SWAN

The morning of the day it was announced to the world that the terrible virus had been categorized as a pandemic, I stood in a lecture hall before 230 students introducing the next unit on the syllabus I had designed months before: apocalyptic narratives. I was teaching a course called Literature and the Environment. The course began with unpacking ideas about what wilderness was exactly and who had access to this wilderness. And we had talked about how to connect with the nonhuman world and the ethics of speaking for nature, the ways in which nature in literature had symbolized human desires and values. And we had reached the point in the course when we would focus on authors who wrote about environmental destruction and human folly. We would begin thinking about why imagining the end of the world was something many writers utilized. Why did humans want to imagine our own demise? What lessons could we take away from these stories? The book I would be teaching followed a solitary sunburned survivor through a postapocalyptic world which had clearly suffered from the effects of severe climate change and had just been decimated by a man-made virus. "See you Monday."

That afternoon, the pandemic was announced. Our classes moved online.

To say that I felt uncomfortable about this would be an understatement. What kind of a professor would continue teaching such a dark book in a moment when students were facing a real catastrophic historical moment?

I considered my options as I learned the tools of teaching at my computer at home. I moved back and forth between reading the terrifying death toll, the constantly evolving rules for avoiding the virus, and tutorials on how to share Word documents with my students as I recorded my voice giving a lecture. I was filled with the desire to present an optimistic, strong persona to my students, but the truth is I was frozen with anxiety.

We learned it was okay to take walks. Taking walks through my neighborhood or by the small lake not far from my house always helps clear my mind. But it seemed different. So few cars were on the roads. The sounds of the winged things dominated the air rather than the sounds of traffic. And was it the urgency I felt to find hope that made me notice so many more birds or was it true there were more this year? I started keeping track of the sightings as though each one was a sign: great blue heron, pileated woodpecker, Baltimore oriole, green heron, rose-breasted grosbeak, wood duck, mourning dove, goldfinch, and even on one rare day, two indigo buntings in my backyard. The world was strewn with jewels. They had made it through the winter. They had migrated through storms, and here they were, continuing. Resilient and beautiful. I thought I would remind my students to go outside and look around.

On one of these walks, I noticed an abandoned nest at the edge of the sidewalk. Nests never fail to impress me. The ingenious architecture, the variety of building materials, the fact that birds built these without hands or blueprints. I picked it up and examined it. The thinnest, softest grasses woven together formed the inside cup of the nest where the baby birds would have huddled together. The outer walls were made first of thicker, longer field grasses and then twigs, which was typical. But this nest had some surprises. Wound into the outermost layer were a long piece of ripped plastic, a narrow strip of metal screen from some abandoned screen door, I imagined, and finally dried hydrangea blossoms. I understood then the message I needed most in this moment. Here was resourcefulness, flexibility, and adaptation.

Birds living in our midst as cities replaced forests had learned how to incorporate bits of our built environment into their lives. Using something like plastic or metal screen was most likely not ideal to the bird's mind, but she used what she had. And she had even added flowers at the end, made her nest beautiful. I needed to keep this in mind as I moved forward in my teaching and in my life.

My students responded so gracefully to the changes we needed to make. They showed up when I went live online. They wrote deeply engaged responses to each other. Still I was worried about the novel. Would it depress them? Scare them? What they found in the book, instead, was a chance to look at the damaging patterns we had created in society. The book looked hard at us and our ability to lose our sense of empathy. As the world paused, they looked deeply into how they wanted things to change when it started up again. How they wanted to build something new and beautiful as they connected to each other and the world.

These students and the birds became my teachers, and my persona of optimism became authentic. Here was the hope I needed.

Heather Swan is the author of the award-winning nonfiction book *Where Honeybees Thrive* and a collection of poems, *A Kinship with Ash*. She teaches writing and environmental literature at the University of Wisconsin-Madison.

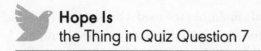

Hope Is
the Thing in Quiz Question 7

KEN SZYMANSKI

For the latest in a long line of quarantine distance-learning assignments, my eighth-grade students listened to an episode of *This American Life*. In the story, a nine-year-old girl bombards her father with the biggest questions in the universe: *Where do we go when we die? Is heaven another planet? How do you know what is true?* And so on.

After listening to the story, students logged into an online quiz. It started with fact recall and then became more abstract. The final question—quiz question 7—echoed the one that the dad in the story had the hardest time answering: what is love?

This question was my student teacher's suggestion. I was skeptical. If I had been asked "What is love?" in eighth grade, I would have responded, "How am I supposed to know?" Plus, the novelty of distance learning had worn thin. Jaded students were no longer giving their all with these ungraded supplemental assignments; I didn't imagine they were eager to dig into such a complex question. Sometimes it felt like these assignments were simply an item to cross off a list, something in the way of them getting on with their days.

Trying to create something more personal, I've been recording and sending the students a series of fake radio call-in shows based on the assignments. I actually added a laugh track after my jokes, to make it sound less lonely.

When I opened the quiz responses and got to quiz question 7, the first student had written a quick "I don't know." Others, though, dove in deep. Some answers were so profound that I put them in a Google search to see if they had gotten that answer online. (A couple did.) But some of these eighth graders, perhaps because of the story or the extended isolation, had turned into sages and philosophers.

Unlike the dad in the story who struggled to answer the "What is love?" question, eighth graders wrote of putting someone before yourself, seeing beyond the façade, and a sense of belonging that "keeps you sane."

One student wrote, "Love is not giving up. It's more than just a word; it's a feeling, it's something you show. Love is something that lingers on your brain even when you don't know it's there."

Another student offered one idea from each side of his brain: "Love could be something purely chemical. Its purpose is keeping our species alive. Or it's something of magic. Magic powerful enough to bind people together. You choose which one you believe in."

I can't imagine formulating those thoughts when I was in eighth grade. I'd have been more like this student who took a comical approach, simply writing, "Kevin Love is a player for the Cleveland Cavaliers."

While some took it lightly, others explored potential perils. One extended answer ended with, "Love can make you feel whole, but it also can break you down until you are nothing."

Another only saw the dangers, simply stating that love is pain.

That's undeniable. Still, some chose to see beyond pain and even, in the case of one student, beyond our physical existence. She listened to the story with her mom and admitted that they both cried. Yet this teenager took solace in the idea that "energy is neither created nor destroyed. And so that's why when someone dies, we can still feel their energy even though they're not there."

That's love, "something that lingers on your brain even when you don't know it's there." And the unwavering belief in it, voiced from quarantined middle schoolers—the next generation—is something more.

It is hope.

Ken Szymanski is a native of Eau Claire, where he lives with his wife and two sons. He teaches English at DeLong Middle School and is the Eau Claire writer-in-residence for 2020–2022.

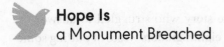

Hope Is
a Monument Breached

SAHAR MAHMOUD TAMAN

June 1, 2020, is a hot, sticky day in Richmond, Virginia. Bisco is taking me for a walk. We do our usual tour down Grace Street, a few blocks from Virginia Commonwealth University at the junction between student apartments and the stately brownstone homes of the city's residents. I am wearing my new cotton mask, handmade by a friend. It's a good one with a nosepiece and a carbon filter.

It's one week after George Floyd was killed by that policeman in Minneapolis. Black Lives Matter protests are starting to swell in this former capital of the Confederacy. The protestors are young people, done with structural racism. I come to Richmond often to see my daughter. I am an intermittent summer Wisconsinite, but this summer I need to be closer to her. I hope to help her overcome the disappointment of her canceled graduation ceremony, a collateral of the coronavirus pandemic.

Grace Street is parallel to Monument Avenue with its infamous confederate monuments that are a lightning rod of the BLM movement. The ostentatious homes on Monument Avenue are well-tended histories as in-your-face reminders of the wealth and power of the Confederate South. Bisco would rather walk Monument Avenue and at every corner turns towards it. He enjoys the larger abundance of flora spilling forth from the superbly kept gardens. He is always hopeful I will let him off the leash to run the grass median, the width of a regular street by itself. When he pulls towards the avenue this time, I follow. There's an 8 p.m. curfew ordered by the governor, a militant response to the protests. Tonight will be the third night of protests. I know the police and the National Guard are getting ready to do something. My hope is that Bisco can enjoy his walk because we won't be able to go again before curfew starts.

I swallow as I head to the statue. I am always bewildered when I see these gargantuan monuments celebrating the legacy of human captivity. Bisco is a black-mouth cur, a breed from the South. He is not bewildered. He loves the smells around the base of the sixty-foot statue. That's where he usually wants to do his doggy business.

As we step on to Lee Circle, ironically mapped as the center of Richmond, I do a double take. I have never seen the Robert E. Lee look so magnificent. The graffiti—"BLM," "Blood on Your Hands," "One Love," and four-letter epitaphs against police cruelty—now define the bastion. Protestors are reclaiming their city. I was here during the August 2017 protests in Richmond, after the Charlottesville white supremacist furor. Then the Lee monument was heavily guarded by police. There was no graffiti then. It could not be breached.

Yet, now I have hope that these monuments will finally go down. Tears flow. I feel the enormous relief of a decade of yearning. For years, I have written to Virginia legislators that these confederate relics are part of the everyday racism that Black communities endure, and that the only option was to melt them to bronze. My hope is that this is now possible.

Bisco is excited as we cross onto the lawn. I enjoy the new art up close. Bisco sniffs the fresh paint. He pulls up his leg and does his business. His hope is fulfilled.

We walk the last two blocks home quickly. A young woman tells me that protestors are headed to the monument, "Like thousands." Later at the apartment, we hear the chants, then shouting, then screams. Bisco jumps onto the couch and barks out the window. I see an armored tank with a National Guardsman atop drive by. After a few minutes, I see protestors running down our street, covering their faces, gasping, crying, angry at the police. The aftermath of tear gas floats outside and seeps under our front door. Bisco gags at the odor until it dissipates. Late into the night, Twitter tells us that at 7:40 p.m., before curfew, Richmond police deployed tear gas and pepper spray at the Lee monument. My heart sinks, but only a little. I still have hope. The protestors will return. Because, this time, the monument was breached.

Sahar Mahmoud Taman grew up in Chippewa Falls and is now an intermittent summer Wisconsinite. She is a mom, law student, Arab Muslim person of color, and a lifelong advocate for social justice.

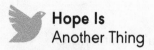

Hope Is
Another Thing

BRUCE TAYLOR

that might not
arrive today but
is on the way
maybe tomorrow

not the edge
you teeter on
but a ledge you
must step off of

a promise made
if as yet unkept
the stark fact of
the always possible

trusting to trust
believing in belief
having faith in faith
hope against hope

Bruce Taylor, professor emeritus, University of Wisconsin-Eau Claire, is former poet laureate of Eau Claire, curator of Local Lit for *Volume One*, and host of the reading series Off the Page. He is author of eight collections of poetry and editor of numerous anthologies.

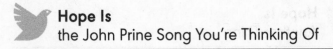

Hope Is
the John Prine Song You're Thinking Of

BEN THEYERL

I was standing in a field in Eau Claire a few years ago when John Prine wandered back into my life. He was playing the Eaux Claires Music & Arts Festival, but I couldn't have told you that while walking down from the parking lot to attend the festival that day. Though twenty-two thousand music lovers from around the world were expected to descend upon Eau Claire, I was only there because a friend offered me a ticket in exchange for parking cars for a few hours with the Knights of Columbus. You know, locals' discount. My friend and I were standing at the foot of the main stage, biding the hours before the headliner—a young Chicago hip-hop artist called Chance the Rapper—was going to take to the stage, when an elderly man with a crooked neck, a crooked smile, and a guitar approached a microphone. His voice was dusty, his music gravelly, and as if those adjectives could become material things, I found myself transported back to traveling a hot, dusty road in the back seat of my grandfather's truck. I remembered how my grandfather had searched the radio airwaves north of Milwaukee, eventually breaking through the radio fuzz to hear a man named John Prine sing "Hello in there, hello." Ten years later, here was that same musician singing that same song on the stage directly before me.

Ever since that moment, I've been processing life via John Prine. Heck, I've been processing this pandemic via John Prine. That's the one comfort to take from John Prine's departure, that others may now know the companionship of his music as well. You could tap Prine as a master at every little thing he did with folk music—from his storytelling, to his wit—but you'd be better off not breaking down his power into pieces. Prine's power was the convergence of those pieces. He did what the best lyricists do: took the world's most complex problems, boiled them down, and showed them to us simply.

Prine's words are poetry, not in the sense that they're so good they're poetry (though they are), but in that they cast shadows and ultimately can be heard and misheard. I will never be an old woman, and I'm not named after my mother, as is the character in his beloved "Angel from Montgomery." But I can tell you that I've asked the same question that character asks: "How the hell can a person go to work in the morning, come home in the evening, and have nothing to say?" Prine shares stories of lives led that we find ourselves leading. His project is giving voice to the human emotions we all feel, no matter our various paths toward reaching them.

This is handy, given our current moment. John Prine never wrote a song about the COVID-19 pandemic. Sadly, he left us before penning a line perfectly articulating the world of self-isolation and stay-at-home orders. There's no Prine song with a nurse character seamlessly wavering between humor and tragedy in caring for their patients to help us remember the specific acts of humanity this time requires. We are left only with sketches. This body of work does insist on one thing, though: hope conquers all other human emotions.

But hope isn't all John Prine gave us. He gave us wisdom, too—wisdom he'd accrued over a lifetime of experiences. While some of his most celebrated work was written during his youthful twenties and thirties, we can't overlook the later years. Prine seemed to slip into old age like he was always meant to be there. He became a caricature of the wise-cracking relative; only when Prine made the joke, he slapped your soul instead of your knee. His music always reached deeper, was more generous. And he proved, song after song, that humor mixed with life equals empathy.

Why did John Prine write songs? As he once put it, because "no one told me I couldn't." Perhaps that's his lasting lesson for those of us stuck here on earth. No one's told us we can't be there for each other, and that we can't be kind, and that we can't be human. And so, we may as well be.

Smoke that nine-mile cigarette, John, and take in the show.

Ben Theyerl is a student and writer from Altoona, Wisconsin, who currently resides in Maine.

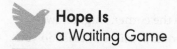

Hope Is
a Waiting Game

ALEX TRONSON

At the supermarket, two men claw each other over a six-pack of toilet paper rolls. They're fighting over the good stuff, though. The off-brand rolls stay stocked, undesired, the last kids picked in gym class. The men are loud. I can hear the fight from my small apartment balcony—the only fresh air I get these days. I retreat inside. This is March. Each time the world ends, I try not to think about it.

I wrestle with the remote and bypass the news for something more my speed, more uplifting. A Bogart film, an episode of *Ghost Adventures*, whatever's popular on HBO. I watch television until my eyes dry up. My partner, Cheryl, is doing taxes in the bedroom. She says to herself, "It all feels kind of futile, now, doesn't it?"

"What does?" I say. "Taxes?"

But she's not talking to me. She's plugged in, crunching numbers and despairing over the sum.

I should be more productive, I think. *Surely, all this time inside could be better utilized. I should write a song or a poem or something.* But then I read on Twitter that we shouldn't feel too bad for not being productive. That we shouldn't feel like we're wasting time. Everyone's coping after all. So, the television continues to strobe.

Deep down, my hope is that someone, somewhere, is working harder than I am. That someone, somewhere is intelligent and qualified and making great leaps of progress. That they aren't feeling as defeated as I am. But hope is easily replaced by anxiety and now I'm cowering by the armchair in the corner. I'm peeking out the window and passing small judgements on the people still wandering around down below.

Later, Cheryl rummages through the pantry. She says, "We should go to the store soon, probably, don't you think?"

"Is that a good idea?" I say from the corner. "Right now?"

"All right," she says. "Fine. How many slices of toast do you want?"

I'm not a scientist. I'm not swabbing the nostrils of the sick or developing vaccine trials. I don't know understand much about health care or sanitation. I'm no parent or caretaker. I'm a grad student. I'm watching old movies and arguing with my friends on the internet. I'm reading thousands of tweets and hardly writing them.

"Do you think we should be doing more?" I say. "Sewing masks and whatnot?"

Cheryl brings over two plates of toast. She sits on the couch, takes a bite and chews it slowly. "You don't know how to sew," she says finally. "Plus, we're inside. We're distant. We're doing what they told us to do. It's a waiting game."

"Is it?" I say. "A waiting game?"

Cheryl shrugs as if to say: what else?

I'm still ducked in the corner. I'm staring out at the sidewalk with shiny, pleading eyes. Cheryl pats the cushion next to her. I climb up on the couch. Her leg rests over my leg. We're alone together—like the ad says on television. But even that is a luxury.

Alex Tronson lived, worked, and studied in Eau Claire before moving to Louisiana to continue his studies as an MFA candidate at the University of New Orleans.

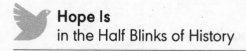

Hope Is
in the Half Blinks of History

ANGIE TRUDELL VASQUEZ

In Light, Always Light

Grass strands gleam weave, undulate from the window

The vendor screams *build the wall*
lifts his hands works the crowd
looks at me   sells more t-shirts.

My mind waxes. Brilliant wet glass winks, waves shine back
    my reflection.

I am dazzled by the sun glinting off my cat's whiskers. He lays
on his back, flanks splayed by the deck   half-shade, half-light.

First graders play football on marigold carpet in our shared
    back yard.
The smile on their faces when they catch it warms us—
childless apartment dwellers behind glass walls.

The poet reads a book of poems then walks to the park to think.
She does not know what she is going to do   hike
the sled hill or swing on the swing. If no children are present
she will swing until her stomach says no, then descend
from her height among the treetops and head home.
She circles the preserve full of earth thoughts: falling leaf
music, crashing, crushing sounds and auburn smells
float up from her footsteps.

She thinks.

We spin on Earth's axis   half-blinks of history.

Angie Trudell Vasquez, a second- and third-generation Mexican American from Iowa, serves on the Wisconsin Poet Laureate Commission. In 2020, she became Madison's first Latina poet laureate.

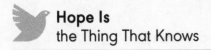

Hope Is
the Thing That Knows

JODI VANDENBERG-DAVES

Hope is the thing that knows
What we cannot know.

It's a pandemic spring in Wisconsin.
The floods came last time the earth spun this way,
And they receded.
The political apocalypse arrived years ago now,
smudging all that we had written.
Nothing was engraved, it turns out.
Change exposes all that we thought we knew.

I feel the soft earth under my feet this morning
On the marsh running trail.
Yesterday the earth felt so vulnerable.
Now, as a scourge of death and disease
Passes among us humans,
The earth resonates like a solid home.
Away from the sidewalks and streets
A bed of sticks and dormant grass holds me up.

Throaty voices of geese pierce the grey and insist on spring.
Bold blue jay's colors shout against the misty, distant sun.
Snow is forced back by warm circles of tree trunks.
Ice is mottled, ridged, patched, thin and fraying
Or thick and angry white-grey, riddled with snow.

And then it's water and the sky is kissing it,
Sharp red lines of leafless bushes line the water's edge,

Vines curlicue up and around sister trees.
Everything is embracing everything else.
What do we ever know about who or what is fragile?

Jodi Vandenberg-Daves is a professor at the University of Wisconsin-La Crosse and the author of *Modern Motherhood: An American History*, various other academic publications, and a self-published collection of poetry, *Poems in the Mother Tongue*.

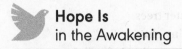

Hope Is
in the Awakening

LISA VIHOS

Once upon a time, the world was falling apart. It had been falling apart for a long time, but too many people were too caught up in their addictions to see it. People had lost sight of themselves and their true purpose: to love one another and protect the Earth.

One day, a terrible disease fell upon the land. Simply being near other people became deadly. Children could not go to school. Adults could not go to work. Choirs could not sing.

When the world shut down, people stopped driving, planes stopped flying, and the first sign of change was that the air got cleaner. The tops of the highest mountains became visible again after years of being shrouded in clouds of pollution.

But on the ground, the virus was spreading. Brave warriors donned masks and set to work on the front lines in hospitals, in factories, in grocery stores. The rest stayed home and loved their families. They baked bread, cleaned their closets, and cut their own hair. Everyone hoped for relief.

When the world shut down, people slowed their pace and began to rethink priorities, to recognize what was truly valuable in their lives. At the brink of losing everything—including life itself—people were aware that they had become aware. They felt as if they had awakened from a bad dream.

A fearful few took their guns to the state house to demand that the world reopen. They were misguided in their denial, because every day, more people got sick. Every day, massive numbers of people died lonely, miserable deaths.

Then one day, George Floyd, a Black man, had his life brutally stolen from him by a white police officer. With that senseless killing, all the racial injustices that had been perpetrated for generations were brought into unmistakably sharp focus. White people—who had refused to look before—had to see. There could be no more turning away.

That murder shed light on so many other Black lives that had been stolen. People of all colors joined forces in the streets, shouting through their masks: "Say Their Names," "No Justice, No Peace, No Justice, No Peace," "Silence is Violence," and "They Can't Breathe."

What became clear was that the dark times had not come from the virus. The dark times had already been present, the result of a world out of balance in every way: racial injustice, the economy, health care, education, the environment, spirituality, everything. Everything was already dark, but those with privilege had turned away. The time came when turning away was no longer an option.

The prophets say a new world will emerge on the other side of COVID-19. Just know, it won't appear magically. People will need to build a better future, working together as one family to end racism, create peace, stand for justice, and protect the Earth; one seed, one poem, one song, one outstretched hand at a time. That is the hope. That, the reality.

The poems of **Lisa Vihos** have appeared in numerous poetry journals, both print and online. She has published four chapbooks and in 2020 was named Sheboygan's first poet laureate.

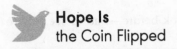

Hope Is
the Coin Flipped

ANGELA VORAS-HILLS

My mother has always loved a good party, and she's great at putting them together. We'd gather for birthdays with platters of taco dip and slow cookers full of beef for sandwiches. She'd throw a baby shower or wedding shower and coordinate games, prepare food, unfold tables and chairs, and fill glass bowls with pastel mints. Mostly, my mom loves to be around people and loves to see them happy.

A few weeks into the COVID-19 Safer at Home order in Wisconsin, my mom called my brother and me from her oncologist's office. She was diagnosed with breast cancer six years ago—six months after my daughter was born, five days after her mother was buried, right after Mother's Day. She went through a series of treatments, and we threw a party when her cancer went into remission. A year later, a routine scan showed the cancer had spread to her liver. She started the fight all over again—labs, chemo, office visits, shrinking tumors, growing tumors. And now she sat alone with her oncologist, both of them in masks, as he tried to talk to us via speaker phone.

Hope is not foolish—I know my mother will die, just as we all will. But I catch myself hoping she'll be here next Christmas, next Easter, my next birthday. It feels greedy to hope so much, so often. We're fortunate she felt well enough during treatment to make new memories—she took her kids and grandkids to Disney World, we all traveled to Texas, she's been able to attend birthday parties, to come to my first book launch. I'm grateful for every good minute she has been able to spend with us. If hope is one side of a coin, the other side is gratitude, and I have a piggy bank full of it.

The oncologist explained the tumors are growing. There's one more treatment, a trial, but he also said it's time to start thinking about hospice, and as long as we're cautious, my mom should be with family now. Days after that call, my mom moved in with my brother and his family, and we created a social bubble. As the weather warmed up, we started getting together to let the kids play outside. Our visits involve a lot of sanitizer, soap, and disinfectant wipes, but it's worth it to see the kids laugh and have fun, and to have my mom around to enjoy these days of sunshine with us.

Earlier this year, my mom planned her funeral. We've talked about visitation and mass, who will bring up the gifts, who will read. She picked a burial plot near her grandmother and designed her own gravestone. My mother loves to plan things, loves when everyone comes together. My hope now is that she'll outlive this pandemic, that this gathering will go according to plan—that we'll get to surround her one last time with everyone she loves.

Angela Voras-Hills's debut poetry collection *Louder Birds* was awarded the Lena-Miles Wever Todd Poetry Prize. She grew up running through fields and forests of Up North, Wisconsin, and currently lives with her family in Milwaukee.

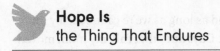

Hope Is
the Thing That Endures

JAMIE VUE

I am a worst-case-scenario, catastrophic-thinking kind of person, but hope is never a memory too far out of reach.

One image comes to mind. My grandmother buoyed by two plastic bags floating across the Mekong River, one tied to each arm to keep her above the murky waters, stiffly holding on for miles before reaching the refugee camps of Thailand.

Four decades later, and she is nearly a century old, if not already. She is the vital element that inspires hope throughout the generations.

But amid the COVID-19 pandemic, some politicians have been entertaining the idea of saving the economy over human lives, offering up the older and elder generations.

I am a byproduct of two cultures, one in which the sacrifice of life was given in the name of freedom, and one that is now considering the sacrifice of life for greed. Deep in my bones I know what it means to be birthed out of an honorable sacrifice. To know an entire generation was devastated, lives lost, so that the younger generations could dream beyond the days of war. That is hope that sustains me. That is hope that a virus can't outlive.

But to snuff out the light of our elders, that doesn't resonate with me.

Growing up, on some days, my parents survived on less than a few dollars with six kids. It is possible. Times were not easy, but we look back on it as a tiny fraction of our lives that taught us some big lessons.

It seems a lifetime ago when my siblings and I were sharing a pack of uncooked ramen noodles, as if breaking bread on the kitchen floor. Now in self-isolation we catch up over virtual chats on the weekends as the nieces and nephew run around in the background. We share photos of our favorite dishes. We clink beers through a computer screen. The six of us once at each other's throats now closely bonded by the times we have survived together. Hope was hard to imagine as kids, but it must have planted itself within us, an intrinsic antidote to the hard times we would face later in life as adults.

Now the children are watching. And one day when they are older, they may need to rely on the history we create for a semblance of hope. And I know that while we are divided in some ways, they will find it in the compassion we give to others. In the lives we save. Because if given a fighting chance, it is likely that people will not give up on themselves.

Jamie Vue is a writing coach at the University of Wisconsin-Stout. She was born in Detroit and attended college in Eau Claire, where she has been living with her husband for the past fifteen years.

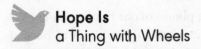

Hope Is
a Thing with Wheels

LARRY WATSON

When I was a boy, I wanted a bicycle. And not just any bicycle but a three-speed Schwinn Corvette, electric blue with white-wall tires and the distinctive Schwinn double crossbar and bi-colored seat. I hoped I'd get that bike, though since I had no reasonable expectation that I'd receive it—I already had a bike, a serviceable one-speed with balloon tires, rattling fenders, and a chain that sometimes slipped—it would probably be more accurate to say I wished for that Schwinn. I would have prayed for it, but I'd already learned, at church and at home, that we were not supposed to pray for selfish purposes or material objects.

Time passed, and I didn't get that bicycle, and while that disappointment wasn't entirely responsible for my realization that nothing comes of hoping, wishing, or praying, it did coincide more or less with my reaching that age when illusions typically begin to drop away. Santa Claus was among the first to fall, but soon to follow were my belief in the unfailing wisdom of parents, teachers, and other elders; the unassailable rightness of my country; the inviolability of the family; the certainty of justice; the permanence of love; even the existence of God.

The cynicism that followed the rejection of naïvely held beliefs was fun for a while—I was young, and it suited a kind of world-weary pose I affected at the time—but cynicism can easily lapse into despair. Even I could see the consequences of life in that state, both for myself and for everyone else on the planet.

But here's the thing. Although I might have believed that hope makes nothing happen, I didn't stop hoping (or wishing or, yes, even letting a prayer sneak out occasionally). I hoped he wouldn't succumb to cancer, I hoped my expression of love would be returned, I hoped the war would end, I hoped that justice would be restored. . . . The specifics weren't as important as the feeling. I still hoped. Perhaps I didn't have the temperament for pessimism.

I wasn't sure—and I'm still not—whether hope breeds optimism or optimism breeds hope, but I could see they worked together. And there I had it—hope alone makes nothing happen. But pair hope with will, with purpose, couple hope with courage, with compassion, and doctors and scientists continue to search for—and discover—treatments and cures for disease, people march for justice and peace, artists produce work that gives pleasure, and we all try to find and create a little more love in our lives. None of this happens without believing that a future is possible when we'll be able to breathe without worrying we're harming ourselves or others, when we can embrace visitors in our homes, when we can pray shoulder to shoulder with fellow congregants, when we can appreciate art in a museum, theater, or concert hall.

That's my hope. And my faith.

Larry Watson is the author of eleven books, including the novel *Let Him Go*, which was made into a movie starring Diane Lane and Kevin Costner. He taught at the University of Wisconsin–Stevens Point for twenty-five years and now lives in Kenosha with his wife.

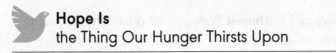

Hope Is
the Thing Our Hunger Thirsts Upon

RACHEL WERNER

Hope is the thing
our hunger thirsts upon.
Despite doubt,
                despair,
                        and ourselves
—most of all.

The pride of man,
responds to Ego's call.
A seductive lure
—enclosing hearts—
behind stonewalls.

We deny Hope's gifts,
to our detriment.
Undeterred, she returns—
a benevolent savior,
in the end.

Feasting upon Joy;
humbled by Folly.
Empathy feeds us,
is the morale—
of Humanity's story.

Rachel Werner is guest faculty for Hugo House and The Loft Literary
Center; a We Need Diverse Books program volunteer; and a book re-
viewer for Shelf Awareness. A Madison resident, she is committed to ho-
listic wellness and sustainable agriculture.

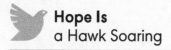

Hope Is
a Hawk Soaring

PETER WHALEN

Hawk hovers over the Boost Mobile burning
on the corner of Locust Street and Dr. Martin
Luther King Way. Smoke pirouettes defy gravity.
Pigeons poke around the curb.

Hawk swoops, flexes feathers.
Skins a pigeon. Checks the weather.
Hawk flies over community elders, who
protect backline marchers.

Hawk knows this land is fed
with lead and asbestos, wells of arsenic,
polluted air and acid rain. Hawk shies
from gunshots and other man-made things.

Perched high on the Sherman Phoenix—
once a burnt-out bank,
now a Black-owned, business hub—
Hawk hears a poet named Hope lead the rally.

Hawk spies their banners.
Hawk watches streets fill with marchers,
who kneel to block the blue. Tires screech.
Car horns scare.

Pigeons peck in a dandelion patch.
Hawk lights for fresh air.

Peter Whalen is a published poet and freelance journalist who currently
teaches English and creative writing at Milwaukee High School of the
Arts. He is the former editor-in-chief of The Cream City Review and education coordinator at Woodland Pattern Book Center in Milwaukee.

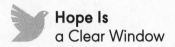

Hope Is
a Clear Window

PETER WHITIS

Many of the stories emerging from this imposed social isolation are of people crammed together. This is the other side of that.

My wife of sixty-seven years is confined to her room at her nursing home due to shelter-in-place coronavirus restrictions. The isolation, everyone required to wear masks, the absence of touch, and the anxiety and sense of solitary confinement were overwhelming her. Her confusion mounted and she had brief periods of panic. I could no longer visit.

Our solution was to meet at the window to her room and talk through our iPhones. We both remembered the time when our third son, Matthew, was born in San Diego during a Santa Ana, a severe dust storm. The San Diego hospital closed to all visitors and our solution was to find a window to her room and visit that way. It wasn't a dust storm grinding into our face this time but an invisible virus invading our community. My wife and I, in our mid-eighties, were deemed especially vulnerable.

After several days of frustrated communication due to a screen that blocked clear vision, Denny, the maintenance chief, came out to see me at the window. He said he could fix that.

The next day he had removed the screen and placed it on another window. He also succeeded in rearranging her room furniture so that she could get closer to the good window. Now we could clearly see one another, and the solitary confinement no longer seemed so devastating.

Hope is a clear window.

Peter R. Whitis, MD, is a retired child psychiatrist who moved with his wife, Martha, to Eau Claire in 2005. His interests are writing, engaging in social activism, playing cribbage, reading, and attending family events.

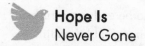

Hope Is
Never Gone

JAKE WRASSE

Hope is never gone, even in the face of an unexpected crisis.

A crisis commands our attention. Even with the worries, fears, and anxieties that we've felt rippling through our culture these past few years, the past few months and COVID-19 have topped everything. The day's headlines threaten to extinguish what hope we have left. As individuals, and as a species, we worry about what the future holds.

We face a real threat, and we're far from through the woods, yet I cannot help but be optimistic about our future. Despite political and cultural divisions, the novel coronavirus—and debates over how we respond—is bringing us together. Trust me, I am as surprised as anyone that hope has not abandoned me, nor I it.

But consider this: When is the last time all of us had to think about the same thing, all the time? When have the consequences ever been this personal, or this dire? When have we had to collectively—separately but simultaneously—reimagine the world as we know it and make changes to support the most vulnerable among us?

These days, we're rethinking our decisions with an eye toward whether or not we're putting others at risk. We're more aware than ever of whether or not we're in someone else's space. I'm not one to gamble, but I'd wager many of us have washed our hands better and more frequently this spring than we did all of last summer.

The creative and rapid recalculations everyone is going through now cannot help but change us. Humans have always sought certainty and repeatability from our experiences, but the world makes no such guarantee. The COVID-19 pandemic has reminded us that ideas are not "common sense" by their own nature, but because we wished them to be enduring truths. If only wishing made it so. How many unimaginable headlines—things you were sure we'd not see in our lifetimes—have you read this month?

We're going to have to find new ways to make sense of our daily experience and be open to solutions we've never considered before. Some of them will work, and some of them won't. But hope will endure, and we'll take that journey together.

This journey will send ripples across the collective pools of common sense into which we search for certainty and predictability in our lives. It will change our notions of what's possible, and what isn't; what's important to us, and what isn't; and the power of the shared humanity that unites us, versus the ideas that divide us. We'll support each other as we grieve the loss of the year we thought we'd have and emerge knowing what we can achieve when we put each other first.

Humans aren't perfect, and we often make things worse than they have to be. But there are always—always—humans working to make things better for other people. Against all odds, hope does not flee. I don't think the coronavirus can change that.

A native of Durand, Wisconsin, **Jake Wrasse** has been writing, reading, and speaking in the Chippewa Valley for as long as he can remember. He does legislative and community relations for the University of Wisconsin–Eau Claire.

Hope Is
the Thing So Small, You Might Almost Miss It

KARISSA ZASTROW

When I first heard the whispers about COVID-19, I hoped it wouldn't make its way north. But then schools and businesses shut down and cases were reported in my county. I felt as though I was sinking, sucked down, and trapped in quicksand. While I try to find my new normal I have been trying to find the calm in quiet and solitude. As someone who thrives on busy hallways, social interactions, laughter, and events, I have had to dig deep to find the small moments that inspire hope.

I found it in the two-hour conversation for the second night in a row with my youngest sister, whom I haven't talked to in months because we've been "too busy." We laughed until we couldn't breathe, and tears trickled down our cheeks. My heart felt lighter.

I found it watching a robin dance on my lawn two days after the first day of spring and four days after my social isolation started. He didn't fly away as I made my way past him to my front door. I paused for a minute as he hopped toward me and looked into my eyes before chirping. I watched until he flew away—a reminder that freedom will come again soon.

I found it in words. First, in a phone call about my grandfather. I chose to focus on the words "caught early" and "very healthy" rather than "cancer" and "surgery." Next, between the words in my new book allowing me to escape real life for a while and live in a pandemic-free world full of social interaction.

I found it in the texts, phone calls, e-mails, and other messages from coworkers, colleagues, friends, classmates, and family checking in to make sure I am okay while isolating alone. I take these moments to reconnect now that parts of life are on pause.

I found it in a stranger who yelled hello to me through her face mask and from a safe distance—a sign that we have not lost our kindness in the madness.

I found it in a new song that I play as loud as I can. I sing-scream along with the artist as I wander around my house, trying to stay busy and keep my anxious thoughts at bay.

I found it along the riverbank, as I listened to the water rush by and cleanse my soul. Looking up at the sky, I took time to imprint the gradation from orange to pink to purple as the sun set in the distance.

I found it when the sun burst through the clouds after a week of grim, gray days as if exclaiming, "Don't worry! I am still here!" I turned toward the sun, soaked in its warmth, closed my eyes and whispered, "Me too."

Karissa Zastrow is a writer and student affairs professional who resides in Wausau. Karissa's work has also appeared in *Twig* and *Wisconsin's Best Emerging Poets*.

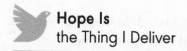

Hope Is
the Thing I Deliver

AMANDA ZIEBA

When I was in middle school I spent an exorbitant amount of time writing notes. Not the studious kind, the tween communication life-line kind. These notes would be written in a rainbow of colors, expertly folded in a complex pattern, and then delivered surreptitiously between classes. Each note was proof of a tangible connection in a sometimes hostile and unpredictable land. I kept the notes I received buried deep in my closet, inside a plastic jug that once held animal crackers. When I left home for college, I threw them away in the name of moving on, but not before unfolding and reading every single one to relive the awkwardly magical times.

In the summer of 2003, I worked at a Bible camp, teaching teenagers about the glory of God while we traveled up and down the Mississippi River on a houseboat. I took the job shortly after breaking up with my first serious boyfriend, though admittedly, by the time I reported to camp, we were back together. Our second-chance romance survived that summer on one phone call a week and lots of letters. Following our second (and final) breakup those letters ended up in the trash. But for that summer the deliveries served as an important tie that held us together.

I shouldn't have been surprised when I returned to letter writing when quarantine rolled around. During the days of the Stay at Home Order, my family and I relied on words to keep our social hearts happy. Each morning, I'd walk out to the mailbox and place in a handful of hope and then put up the little red flag. For months we traded pen-pal letters with friends, sent cards to family members, and drew pictures for classmates.

I am not a health-care worker. Nor can I sew a mask. Or visit my grandfather. Or smile at my coworkers. Or meet for coffee

193

with friends. But the one thing I could do was write letters. I could deliver hope, one stamped envelope at a time.

And here's the thing about hope. It comes back around. For the brief moment it takes to open the door of my mailbox and peer inside I'm uncertain of what I'll find. I'll go days with nothing but bills, but then, just when it seems like the mail service only delivers responsibilities and bad news, a bright envelope shows up, with my name scrawled in recognizable handwriting. Hope.

Amanda Zieba works to help other writers tell their own stories through courses, workshops, and retreats. She lives in Holmen, Wisconsin, with her husband and two sons.

Acknowledgments

Editing a book consisting of one hundred contributors has been described to me as a "leap of faith," "a fool's errand," and, perhaps most memorably, "one gigantic herding of cats." Yet in reality, this book's contributors ensured that it was never anything but a true pleasure.

To begin, a profound thank you to Erika Wittekind, Gary Smith, Kate Thompson, Elizabeth Boone, John Ferguson, and the Wisconsin Historical Society Press for bringing this book to light.

Thank you, too, to my colleagues at the University of Wisconsin–Eau Claire, and in particular Chancellor James Schmidt, Provost Patricia Kleine, President Kimera Way, Dean Rodd Freitag, Dean Carmen Manning, Dr. Jan Stirm, Dr. Justin Patchin, Dr. Jason Spraitz, Dr. Dorothy Chan, and Professors Max Garland, Jon Loomis, Allyson Loomis, Molly Patterson, Bruce Taylor, and John Hildebrand. Thanks to Nick Butler, Patti See, Eric Rasmussen, Ken Szymanski, Andy Patrie, Julian Emerson, Jeff DeGrave, Jim Alf, Steve and Stacey Dayton, and Emily Kubley. The list goes on.

In addition, thank you to Dr. Catherine Chan and the Office of Research and Sponsored Programs at the University of Wisconsin–Eau Claire, whose University Research and Creative Activity grant proved vital to this project.

And finally, to my family, who always encourage me to take the leap, embrace the fool's errand, and herd the cats as necessary. Hope is you.

About the Editor

B. J. Hollars is the author of several books, most recently *Go West Young Man: A Father and Son Rediscover America*, *Midwestern Strange: Hunting Monsters, Martians, and the Weird in Flyover Country*, and *The Road South: Personal Stories of the Freedom Riders*. His work has been featured in the *Washington Post* and *Parents Magazine*, on NPR, and elsewhere. He is the recipient of

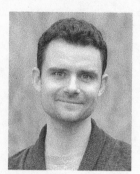

Photo by Brian Hollars

the Truman Capote Prize for Literary Nonfiction, the Anne B. and James B. McMillan Prize, the Council of Wisconsin Writers Blei-Derleth Award, and the Society of Midland Authors Award. Additionally, he is the founder and director of the Chippewa Valley Writers Guild, the Midwest Artist Academy, and The Priory Writers' Retreat, as well as an associate professor of English at the University of Wisconsin–Eau Claire.